CW00521852

Title: The path to Enlightenment from the practice of Tai Chi + Zhàn zhuāng (pile stance)

Sub title: The Shen Ming of Tai Chi is the complementary component of your meditation for Enlightenment

By George Ho
Co-authors: Rebecca Ho, Jennifer Ho
All copyrights reserved

Series Information: tai chi and meditation   3
The abridged version of this article, "The Significance of Dong jin"

was first published in the 2014 Fall issue of T'ai Chi Magazine,

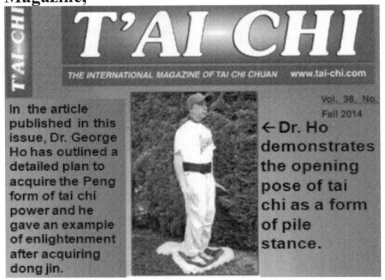

In the article published in this issue, Dr. George Ho has outlined a detailed plan to acquire the Peng form of tai chi power and he gave an example of enlightenment after acquiring dong jin.

← Dr. Ho demonstrates the opening pose of tai chi as a form of pile stance.

copyright-protected by Wayfarer Publications, 2601 Silver Ridge Ave., Los Angeles, CA 90039. All rights including translated versions reserved. No part of this article may be used or reproduced in any manner without written permission of the author, Dr. George Ho, who can be contacted by email: Georgekwho@gmail.com or Georgekwho@yahoo.com.

懂勁 "Dong jin" as the stepping stone into the state of 神明(Shén míng) is taken from A phrase from 王宗岳 Wángzōngyuè's 太極拳論 (tàijí quán lùn;theory of tai chi) , "由(from)著熟(zhe shú; knowing the moves well)而漸悟懂勁。由懂勁 (dong jin; knowing the operation of the 8 forms of tai chi power)而階及神明 (shen ming; getting results in enlightenment and longevity)"

The original 太極拳論 (tàijí quán lùn;theory of tai chi):

太極者，無極而生，陰陽之母也。動之則分，靜之則合。無過不及，隨曲就伸。人剛我柔謂之走，我順人背謂之粘。動急則急應，動緩則緩隨。雖變化萬端，而理爲一貫。**由著熟而漸悟懂勁，由懂勁而階及神明**。然非用力日久，不能豁然貫通焉。虛靈頂勁，氣沈丹田。不偏不倚，忽隱忽現。左重則左虛，右重則右杳。仰之則彌高，俯之則彌深，進之則愈長，退之則愈促。一羽不能加，蠅蟲不能落，人不知我，我獨知人。英雄所向無敵，蓋皆由此而及也。斯技旁門甚多，雖勢有區別，概不外壯欺弱、慢讓快耳。有力打無力，手慢讓手快，是皆先天自然之能，非關學力而有爲也。察四兩撥千斤之句，顯非力勝；觀耄耋禦衆之形，快何能焉。立如秤準，活似車輪，偏沈則隨，雙重則滯。每見數年純功，不能運化者，率皆自爲人制，雙重之病未悟耳。欲避此病，須知陰陽；粘即是走，走即是粘，陽不離陰，陰不離陽；陰陽相濟，方爲懂勁。懂勁後，愈練愈精，默識揣摩，漸至從心所欲。本是舍己從人，多誤「捨近求遠」。所謂「差之毫釐，謬以千里。」學者不可不詳辨焉。是爲論。"

This article covers many topics regarding the concept of 懂勁 "Dong jin" that could lead the practitioners into the enlightenment stage, called 神明(Shén míng) in tai chi and the importance of the acquisition of the CranioSacral postural reflex in Tai Chi.
The abstract of the book:

This article is the enriched version of the article published in T'ai Chi magazine in 2014. It covers many topics regarding the concept of of 懂勁 "Dong-jin (understanding the power of tai chi)" that could lead the practitioners into the Enlightenment stage, called 神明(Shén míng) in tai chi. The importance of the new health concept called the CranioSacral postural reflex in Tai Chi is introduced in this article. The theme of discussion revolves around the following quote from the Theory of Tai Chi by the ancient sage, Wang Zongyue 王宗岳 (around 1771~1853):

"由著熟(Zhe shú, meaning to have known the movements by heart)而漸悟(Wù, comprehend)懂勁 (Dong jin)，由(Yu, from)懂勁(Dong jin) 而階及(step into)神明(Shén míng)，然非用力之久(without a long period of practice)，不能豁然(Huòrán)貫通 (guàntōng)焉(cannot obtain a sudden breakthrough into the state of enlightenment to advance into the 神明(Shén míng) stage。"

My translation of "由著熟(Zhe shú, meaning to have known the movements by heart)而漸悟(Wù, comprehend)懂勁(Dong jin)，由(Yu, from)懂勁而階及 (Jiē jí, step into)神明(Shén míng, enlightenment"):

The chosen tai chi movements have become so well practiced that the practitioner reaches the state of 懂勁 Dong jin, which means that the mind/body complex has established a new and very efficient pathway in the neural system. Using this new mind/body complex as the platform of further refinement might lead to enlightenment coveted by so many practitioners. One of the benign side effects of this new mind/body complex is its health enhancement to release stress with the practice of meditation. 神明(Shén míng) is a very vague term that could have quite a few interpretations. 神(Shén) as a noun means "god". It could be an adjective, meaning miraculous. 明(míng) can be an adjective, meaning "bright" and it can be a verb, meaning "to understand". In the above context, I think Shén míng means a "miraculous" upgrade of intelligence. Shén míng in tai chi is similar to 頓悟 Dùnwù, the sudden emergence of direct knowledge in Chan Buddhism. This will be further elaborated later in this article.

In our modern age after the 2nd World War I have never heard of any tai chi master, who has reached this Shén míng stage of super intelligence, especially when most people practice tai chi as a form of martial arts. Most tai chi practitioners are impressed by masters, who can demonstrate their superior power to push people flying up in the air. This kind of kung fu does not have any practical value in real fighting. It has never appeared in a real fight.

Shen ming in the sense of Enlightenment has a far more significant value in our modern age that values the soul as much as the body. Master Sun Lutang (1860-1933), who emphasized heavily on 站椿 Zhàn zhuāng (pile stance) as the fundamental training of Tai Chi has shown us this possibility of Enlightenment with his martial arts discipline. The following is the report of his Enlightenment in the media in 1933:

Master Sun stunned the world when he ended his life in a Daoist's way of self-administered euthanasia to enter another state of his life, immortality. In his late years, Master Sun Lutang was living in retirement in the countryside; he predicted the day of his death and practiced 辟穀 Bi Gu for two days (for an enlightened Daoist, Bi Gu means eating only a small amount of raw food and eventually to stop eating before his or her spirit leaves the physical body.) When the time came, he sat on a chair in a Confucian manner, facing southwest with his back to the northwest and told the family members not to cry and said to them, "I regard death only as a game." At 6:05 AM in 1933 he died with a smile. The major Chinese newspapers and magazines such as the 《申報》《民國日報》《大公報》《益世報》《世界日報》 reported his special way to die like an enlightened Daoist. All the editorials spoke highly of him. In major cities like Nanjing, Shanghai, Hangzhou, Beijing, and Tianjin many martial arts groups held public memorial services for Master Sun.

Contents:

1/"由著熟(Zhe shú, meaning to have known the movements by heart)而漸悟(Wù, comprehend)懂勁 (Dong jin)，由(Yu, from)懂勁(Dong jin) 而階及(step into)神明(Shén míng)，然非用力之久(without a long period of practice)，不能豁然(Huòrán)貫通 (guàntōng)焉(cannot obtain a sudden breakthrough into the state of enlightenment to advance into the 神 明(Shén míng) stage。" …p.15

2/The following breathing practice is a concrete example of reaching 神明 (Shén míng, enlightenment) in the above quotation. …p.41

3/Between 著熟(Zhe shú, meaning to have known the movements by heart)and 懂勁(Dong jin) Yang Chengfu added 鬆開 "Song kai"..p.59

4/When your body is in a "Song kai" state you can efficiently "store up power like a bow being drawn and release it like a heavily loaded arrow 蓄勁如張弓，發勁如放箭", according to Yǔxiāng Wǔ's (1812-1880) 武禹襄《太極拳解 *Tàijí quán jiě*》. …p.70

5/ After reaching this state of dǒng jìn one's Tai Chi kung fu can improve qualitatively by the continuous practice of the complementary cooperative actions of the yin and the yang. The more one practices the better the Tai Chi dǒng jìn kung fu will become. The original text of the above translation is as followed, "陰 陽 相濟方為懂勁。懂勁後。愈練愈精。" (陰 =yin, 陽=yang, 相濟= complementing each other, 方為懂勁。懂勁後 =after the acquisition of dong jin。愈練愈精 =continuous improvement。.p.71

6/ The most significant mind body enhancement transformation is the state after "懂勁 dong jin", called the 神明 Shén míng state. p.72

7/ I would like to add that many enlightened scholars like 南懷瑾 Nán Huái jǐn went one step further with this tai chi Dong jin level to practice Chan meditation and reached their coveted enlightenment, called 頓悟 Dùn wù in Chan Buddhism. .p.73

8/Any posture as exemplified by all the Buddhist statues is possible for this state to emerge as long as it has the CranioSacral postural reflex of tai chi, the weight-less feeling of the head, called Ding Tou Xuan 頂頭懸 and an adhesive feeling of the abdominal part below the umbilicus, called Qi Tie Bai 氣貼背 when the practitioner feels that the aforementioned anatomical part is sticking towards the spine..p.83

9/Practicing the Nine Sessions Buddhist Wind Breathing,九節佛風 Jiǔ jié fú fēng according to Tibetan Buddhism is one of the ways to reach Shen ming:p.91

10/In another writing of Master Wǔ, "The explanation of the 13 Tai Chi moves 十三勢行功心解 Shísān shì xíng gōng xīn jiě", he said, "Each Tai Chi move is a cycle that should have a total body movement of muscle contraction and relaxation. His original wording is as followed, "往復須有摺疊=folding". The modern concept of alternative muscle contraction and relaxation to store and release power is better visualized by the analogy of a coiled spring instead of an arrow. The coiled spring analogy was used by Master Yǔxiāng Wǔ's contemporary, the Yang style Tai Chi family, in their secret instruction manual of the cultivation of the 8 basic forms of power in Tai Chi …p.100

11/The peng form of power is the first and the most important of the 8 basic forms of power in Tai Chi and these 8 basic forms of power have been vaguely explained in a set of definitions, kept as a top secret by the Yang style Tai Chi family for many years.p.102

12/ My complex translation of the peng form of power is consistent with the water buoyancy of a boat carrying weight. A boat in the water will not forcefully resist any weight added on it. It will give room for the weight and build up just enough resistance to deal with the problem.p.105

13/This kind of connecting the muscles of the total body movements, called the practice of pile standing can be practiced by itself or at the beginning of a Tai Chi practice...p.106

14/This is probably the best and the most integrative way to cure poor posture. This new interpretation opens up some new usages of Tai Chi . It can be used to treat poor posture, which is becoming epidemic with the new computer technology...p.111

15/ The preparatory pose itself can be an effective form of exercise too...p.112

16/ In order to practice dong jin one of the prerequisites is to have acquired the physical condition as described by Master Chengfu Yang 楊澄甫 as "鬆開 Song kai"..p.113

17/The slow Tai Chi set practice plays the role of enhancing and reinforcing the newly learned postural reflex so that it can be maintained during movements...p.115

18/The peng form of power, demonstrated by Dr. George Ho in June, 2014: p.117

19/Because of China's deep cultural influence most Chinese have been somewhat conditioned to think that the traditional or the secret teachings are the guarantee of their success in learning that form of art.p.122

20/I have found that Dantian singing in Chinese opera is another way. It is more objectively observable because the progress in singing and chanting can be easily observed, recorded and compared…p.138

21/I have combined Dantian singing with my Dolphin Instant tai chi when I swim and Treadmill Ram Tai Chi my hiking…p.139

<u>Links used in this article:</u>

https://zh.wikipedia.org/wiki/太極拳論

https://www.youtube.com/watch?v=Za0wxuF4jlg

https://www.youtube.com/watch?v=eTOEjBWFr-8
鄭曼青 - 推手 and the   push hand is at 2.37.

• The Power of Internal Martial Arts and Chi: Combat and Energy Secrets of Ba Gua, Tai Chi and Hsing-I by

• Bruce Frantzis (1949-)

 The link show of the cover of this book is
http://www.barnesandnoble.com/w/the-power-of-internal-martial-arts-and-chi-bruce-frantzis/1111615333?ean=9781583941904

https://www.youtube.com/watch?v=iKwubHzyuFk

The supernatural "direct knowledge" helped Huì néng become the Patriarch of Chan Buddhism

南老师示范九节佛风及宝瓶气 (Eng Sub) ,uploaded by TransparentSeed

https://www.youtube.com/watch?v=ov5ObN82mFowei
Dantian 丹田 manifestation,韻味 Yùnwèi a unique
characteristic in Chinese art including martial art
https://www.youtube.com/watch?v=fe-PoZkQKYI
(1)Tai chi breathing cultivated by Dantian singing as a
form of throat and tongue tai chi
https://www.youtube.com/watch?v=5i0dN9zryQ8
(2)Tai chi breathing cultivated by Dantian singing as a
form of throat and tongue tai chi
https://www.youtube.com/waOJVbymIYjQMtch?v=
"Beyond Relaxation" in tai chi and therapeutic
seminars using tai chi power
https://www.youtube.com/watch?v=LPbKYpoIMEU
The Tai Chi CranioSacral Postural Reflex for better
posture and tai chi (Copyrights reserved)

https://www.youtube.com/watch?v=UbVy Uo16nw4

A supplemental movie to my first article of my Dantian
and Mingmen' series (All copyrights reserved)

Title: "Shen Ming is the Enlightenment Stage of Tai Chi, Superior to the Martial Arts Stages of Song Kai and Dong Jin"

The old title published in the T'ai Chi Magazine in 2014: "In order to benefit and to excel in Tai Chi, Dǒng jìn 懂勁 is crucial"

According to the tai chi classics, 《太極拳論 *Tàijí quán lùn*》 written by Zongyue Wang 王宗岳 (around 1771~1853) 《太極拳論》·山右　*王宗岳 https://zh.wikipedia.org/wiki/太極拳論:

太極者，無極而生，陰陽之母也。動之則分，靜之則合，無過不及，隨曲就伸。人剛我柔謂之「走」，我順人背謂之「粘」，動急則急應，動緩則緩隨，雖變化萬端，而理唯一貫。**由著熟而漸悟懂勁，由懂勁而階及神明，然非用力之久，不能豁然貫通焉....**。

1/"由著熟(Zhe shú, meaning to have known the movements by heart)而漸悟(Wù, comprehend)懂勁(Dong jin)，由(Yu, from)懂勁(Dong jin) 而階及(step into)神明(Shén míng)，然非用力之久(without a long period of practice)，不能豁然(Huòrán)貫通(guàntōng)焉(cannot obtain a sudden breakthrough into the state of enlightenment to advance into the 神明(Shén míng) stage。"

My translation of "由著熟(Zhe shú,meaning to have known the movements by heart)而漸悟(Wù, comprehend)懂勁(Dong jin)，由(Yu, from)懂勁而階及(Jiē jí, step into)神明(Shén míng, enlightenment":

The chosen tai chi movements have become so well practiced that the practitioner reaches the state of 懂勁 Dong jin, which means that the mind/body complex has established a new and very efficient pathway in the neural system. Using this new mind/body complex as the platform of further refinement might lead to enlightenment coveted by so many practitioners. One of the benign side effects of this new mind/body complex is its health enhancement to release stress with the practice of meditation. 神明(Shén míng) is a very vague term that could have quite a few interpretations. 神(Shén) as a noun means "god". It could be an adjective, meaning miraculous. 明(míng) can be an adjective, meaning "bright" and it can be a verb, meaning "to understand". In the above context I think Shén míng means a "miraculous" upgrade of intelligence. Shén míng in tai chi is similar to 頓悟 Dùnwù , the sudden emergence of direct knowledge in Chan Buddhism. This will be further elaborated later in this article. I in our modern age after the 2nd World War I have never heard of any tai chi master, who has reached this Shén míng stage of super intelligence, especially when most people practice tai chi as a form of martial arts. Most tai chi practitioners are impressed by masters, who can demonstrate their superior power to push people flying up in the air.

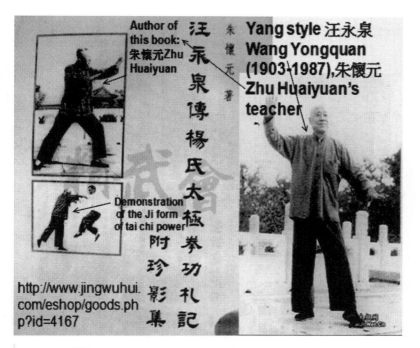

Author of this book: 朱懷元 Zhu Huaiyuan

汪永泉傳楊氏太極拳功礼記附珍影集記

Yang style 汪永泉 Wang Yongquan (1903-1987), 朱懷元 Zhu Huaiyuan's teacher

Demonstration of the Ji form of tai chi power

http://www.jingwuhui.com/eshop/goods.ph p?id=4167

The 擠 Ji power is often used by many famous masters in demonstrations to throw people up in the air as seen in the Youtube video, 鄭曼青- 推手 (A Yang style master, Zhèng Mànqīng – push hand; the link is in the illustrations down below.) at 2.37.

I have seen a lot of injuries from tai chi push hand. In my article I have better ways to train and to evaluate one's tai chi power than to push people.

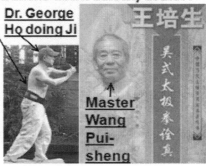

Dr. George Ho doing Ji

王培生

美式太极拳徑真

Master Wang Pui-sheng

This act of demonstrating the Ji form of tai chi power was probably invented by Yang 楊 Shǎo hóu 少侯(1862-1930), the son of the founder of Yang style tai chi, Yang Lu-chan. I do not think it can be used in a real fight and I have never seen it captured in any footage of a real fight either. It can only be performed in demonstrations when the pusher has the cooperation of the person being pushed. In other words, it does not have any real value in combat application.

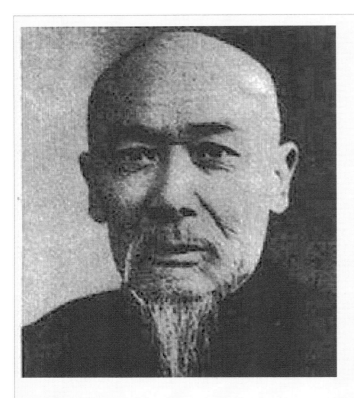

(1862-1930)

https://en.wikipedia.org/wiki/Yang_Shao-hou

Yang 楊 Shǎo hóu 少 侯 taught this demonstration technique to Wang Yongquan (1903-1987) and he taught this to Zhu Huaiyuan(1911-1999).

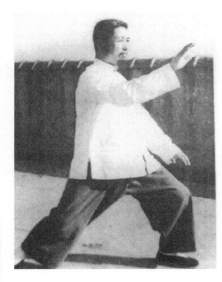

鄭曼青師承楊澄甫,鄭老師是楊家太極第四代代表

Master Man-ching Cheng is the 4th generation representative of the Yang style Tai chi

Chen Man-ching used this in his demonstrations very often to impress people and he became famous in New York in the 60s.

You can watch his demonstration in the following movie onYouTube:

https://www.youtube.com/watch?v=eTOEjBWFr-8
鄭曼青 - 推手 and the push hand is at 2.37.

• The Power of Internal Martial arts s and Chi: Combat and Energy Secrets of Ba Gua, Tai Chi and Hsing-I by

• Bruce Frantzis (1949-) also used this in his book cover:

 The link show of the cover of this book is http://www.barnesandnoble.com/w/the-power-of-internal-martial-arts-and-chi-bruce-frantzis/1111615333?ean=9781583941904

This demonstration of tai chi power that has very little practical combat usage or benefit for health has been valued for over 100 years.

Another useless demonstration is well documented by Dr. Robert C. Sohn who died in 1997 at the young age of 58. He wrote a tai chi kung fu book titled *Tao and T'ai Chi Kung*, published in 1987, by Destiny Books. It is available in the Amazon online bookstore. On the cover is a drawing of his performance the immovable Tai Chi stance, which is substantiated by a photo-picture in p.36, and another photo-picture, described as the unliftable stance in p.38).

I have put together a pictorial description of this demonstration:

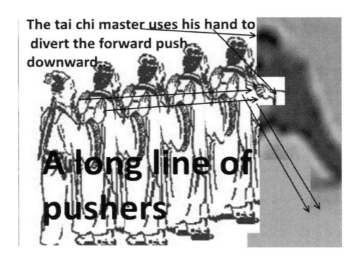

The tai chi master uses his hand to divert the forward push downward.

A long line of pushers

The tai chi master demonstrating this trick uses the first person of that long line of people to redirect all the power downward. Please view this movie in terms of the aforementioned explanations to see for yourself:

https://www.youtube.com/watch?v=vuy1TFgK3EY

太极拳之"千斤坠"，不知道外国人看到这个会相信么？

If YouTube deletes this movie you probably still can watch it in the Chinese internet:

http://www.xizi.tv/txvideos/o0326cjjee8/

This is still being used to impress people and the above demonstration on YouTube occurred in contemporary China because Master 陈 小 旺 Chén Xiǎowàng (1945), a very well-known Chen Style tai chi master appeared in the movie at 3.01 and he used this as a demonstration himself too and the footage is in the Chinese internet.

If this is really useful in resisting a strong push as shown in those demonstrations and it was well demonstrated by Dr. Robert C. Sohn as early as 1987 would it not be adopted in various sports like American Football that pays high prices for players with this kind of super-human talent?

On the other hand if any tai chi practitioner applies the post-dong jin practice time into meditation his or her mental state will gradually improve up to a qualitative turning point of enlightenment of Shen ming, the ulterior goal of the inventor of tai chi as a form of self-refinement. Even before that turning point his or her friends will notice that he or she has become more intelligent in problem solving and has become a better speaker and thinker with quick wits and a keen sense of humour.

In Chinese history there was a Chan (Zen in Japanese) monk that behaved exactly like my above descriptions;

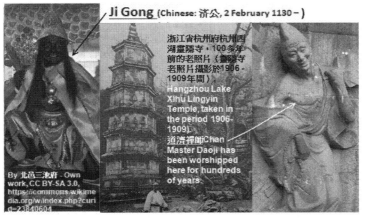

Ji Gong (Chinese: 济公, 2 February 1130 –)

浙江省杭州府杭州西湖灵隐寺，100多年前的老照片（灵隐寺老照片摄影於1906-1909年間）Hangzhou Lake Xihu Lingyin Temple, taken in the period 1906-1909). 道济禅師Chan Master Daoji has been worshipped here for hundreds of years.

By 北邑三漥府 - Own work, CC BY-SA 3.0, https://commons.wikimedia.org/w/index.php?curid=23840604

濟公禪師 Ji Gong (Chinese: 济公, 2 February 1130 – 16 May 1207), born Li Xiuyuan and also known as "Chan Master Daoji" (Chinese: 道濟禪師) was a Chan Buddhist monk who lived in the Southern Song Dynasty. He purportedly possessed supernatural healing powers, which he used to help the poor and stand up to injustice. However, he was also known for his wild and eccentric behaviour and for violating Buddhist monastic rules by consuming alcohol and meat. He knew his supernatural healing ability was unreliable and therefore always denied he had that ability and always pretended he was a crazy monk to hide his real identity. By the time of his death, Ji Gong had become a folk hero in Chinese culture and a minor deity in Chinese folk religion. He is mentioned by Buddhists in folktales and kōans, and sometimes invoked by oracles to assist in worldly affairs.

https://en.wikipedia.org/wiki/Ji_Gong

I have an in-depth explanation of his eccentric behavior at 4.4 minute in my YouTube movie:

https://www.youtube.com/edit?video_id=mrWHuLxQ_ Yw&video_referrer=watch

Sleeping qi gong by Dr. George Ho of Vancouver

Another example of this kind of enlightenment from meditation is Huineng (Chinese: 惠能; pinyin: Huìnéng, 638–713). He was a Buddhist monk who is one of the most important figures in Chan (Zen in Japanese) Buddhism. The following movie on YouTube shows how the supernatural ability of "poem composition by direct knowledge" helped Huineng become the Sixth and the last Patriarch of Chan Buddhism:

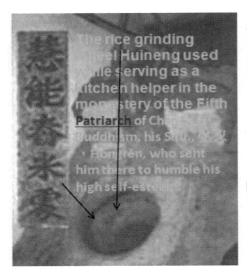

The supernatural ability of " poem composition by direct knowledge" helped an illiterate monk , **Huineng** become the Sixth and the last Patriarch of Chan Buddhism.

https://www.youtube.com/watch?v=iKwubHzyuFk

The supernatural "direct knowledge" helped Huì néng become the Patriarch of Chan Buddhism

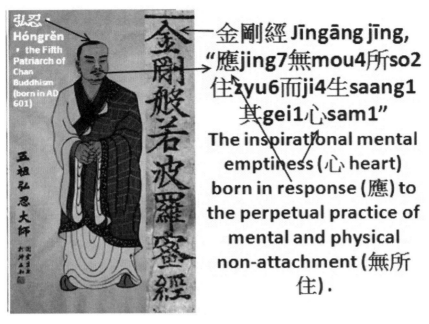

金剛經 Jīngāng jīng,
"應jing7無mou4所so2
住zyu6而ji4生saang1
其gei1心sam1"
The inspirational mental emptiness (心 heart) born in response (應) to the perpetual practice of mental and physical non-attachment (無所住).

In this picture is Huineng's master, Hongren. Hóngrĕn was famous for using the Buddhist script, 金剛經 Jīngāng jīng to teach Chan Buddhism. The illiterate monk, Huineng was never educated. However when he heard this saying in Jīngāng jīng,"應無所住而生其心" My translation of 應無所住而生其心:

The inspirational mental emptiness (心 heart) is born in response (應) to the perpetual practice of mental and physical non-attachment (無所住) .This is very hard for me to imagine how an illiterate monk could get enlightenment so strong that motivated him to travel to a far away province to seek further education from 弘忍，Hóngrěn, who was impressed with 惠能 Huì néng's intelligence and wanted Huì néng to succeed him. Hong ren told all the competing candidates who wanted to be his successor to compose a Chan poem. From the sophistication of the Chan poems he would select his successor. My translation of 惠能 Huì néng's poem, 菩提本無樹，明鏡亦非台；本來無一物，何處惹塵埃？:

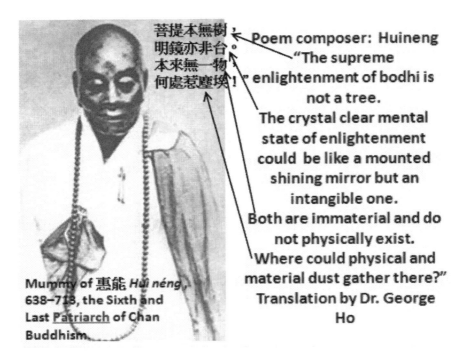

菩提本無樹，
明鏡亦非台。
本来無一物，
何處惹塵埃！

Poem composer: Huineng
"The supreme enlightenment of bodhi is not a tree. The crystal clear mental state of enlightenment could be like a mounted shining mirror but an intangible one. Both are immaterial and do not physically exist. Where could physical and material dust gather there?"
Translation by Dr. George Ho

Mummy of 惠能 Huì néng, 638–713, the Sixth and Last Patriarch of Chan Buddhism.

"The supreme enlightenment of bodhi is not a tree. The crystal-clear mental state of enlightenment could be like a mounted shining mirror but an intangible one. Both are immaterial and do not physically exist. Where could any physical material, like dust gather there?"

To make the long story short, Huineng succeeded by using this "direct knowledge of poem composition", which is one of the lesser forms of supernatural ability, a manifestation of the sophistication of your Chan practice? I have this "supernatural ability of poem composition by direct knowledge" too but I don't know how I got it.

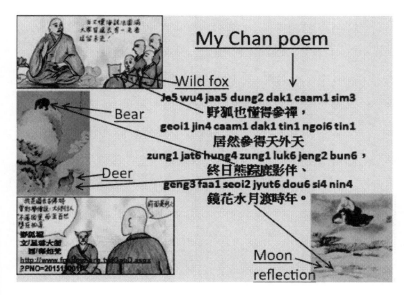

My poem in Mandarin Romanisation:
野狐也懂得參禪，Yě hú yě dǒngde cānchán,
居然參得天外天，jūrán cān dé tiānwài tiān,.
終日熊踪鹿影伴, zhōngrì xióng zōng lù yǐng bàn,

鏡花水月渡時年。 jìnghuāshuǐyuè dù shí nián

The translation of my Chan poem:

This wild fox not only can practice Chan meditation.
He does it with so much dedication that he has reached
the extra superior level above Heaven.
He befriends bears and deer as his companions.
He knows the beautiful scenery surrounding him is just
images as unreal as the reflections of the flowers in the
mirror and the moon shadow on the surface of the lake.
The source of the above poem is from the Wild Fox
Koan:

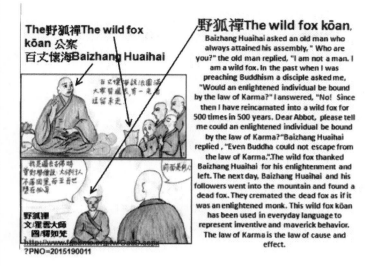

The illustrations in the picture have been enlarged in the following picture:

野狐禪The wild fox kōan.

Baizhang Huaihai asked an old man who always attained his assembly, " Who are you?" the old man replied, "I am not a man. I am a wild fox. In the past when I was preaching Buddhism a disciple asked me, "Would an enlightened individual be bound by the law of Karma?" I answered, "No! Since then I have reincarnated into a wild fox for 500 times in 500 years. Dear Abbot, please tell me could an enlightened individual be bound by the law of Karma?"Baizhang Huaihai replied , "Even Buddha could not escape from the law of Karma.".The wild fox thanked Baizhang Huaihai for his enlightenment and left. The next day, Baizhang Huaihai and his followers went into the mountain and found a dead fox. They cremated the dead fox as if it was an enlightened monk. This wild fox kōan has been used in everyday language to represent inventive and maverick behavior. The law of Karma is the law of cause and effect.

The founder of Chan Buddhism, Bodhidharma 達摩 (440-528) is another good example of wisdom, 慧 Huìin (in Chinese), arisen out of the calm and balanced mental state of meditation, called 定 ding (Samādhi 三昧地) in Chinese.

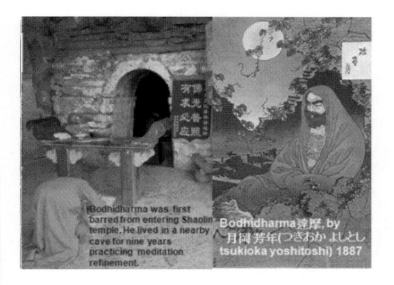

The illustrations in the picture have been enlarged in the following picture:

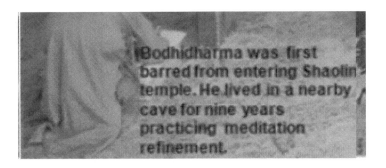

Bodhidharma was first barred from entering Shaolin temple. He lived in a nearby cave for nine years practicing meditation refinement.

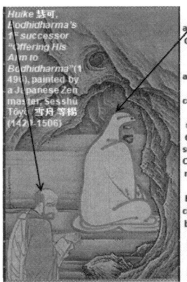

Huike 慧可, Bodhidharma's 1st successor "Offering His Arm to Bodhidharma" (1496), painted by a Japanese Zen master, Sesshū Tōyō 雪舟 等楊 (1420-1506)

Bodhidharma達摩 (440-528) was a Buddhist monk from India. He came to China in the Liang 梁 dynasty (502–557). Bodhidharma was first barred from entering Shaolin temple and was admitted into the temple after nine years of meditation refinement in a nearby cave and he taught there for some time, leaving behind the oral instructions of some Indian yoga, later being named in Chinese as 易筋經 Yì jīn jīng，洗髓經 Xǐ suǐ jīng, which were crossed trained with Chinese martial art by the Shaolin monks, making Shaolin kung fu unique and well-known to the world. In actual fact Bodhidharma's major contribution is his creation of Chan Buddhism, characterised by頓悟 Dùnwù, a sudden enlightenment breakthrough from the practice of 定 dìng, a mental physical state of balance and calmness of thoughtlessness.
https://en.wikipedia.org/wiki/Bodhidharma

The illustrations in the picture have been enlarged in the following picture:

Bodhidharma達摩 (440-528) was a Buddhist monk from India. He came to China in the Liang 梁 dynasty (502–557). Bodhidharma was first barred from entering Shaolin temple and was admitted into the temple after nine years of meditation refinement in a nearby cave and he taught there for some time, leaving behind the oral instructions of some Indian yoga, later being named in Chinese as 易筋經 Yì jīn jīng，洗髓經 Xǐ suǐ jīng, which were crossed trained with Chinese martial art by the Shaolin monks, making Shaolin kung fu unique and well-known to the world. In actual fact Bodhidharma 's major contribution is his creation of Chan Buddhism, characterised by 頓悟 Dùnwù, a sudden enlightenment breakthrough from the practice of 定 ding, a mental physical state of balance and calmness of thoughtlessness.

https://en.wikipedia.org/wiki/Bodhidharma

Very often Shaolin Kung Fu practitioners credit their martial arts' origin to Bodhidharma, who probably did not value the practice of martial arts too much because his main interest is enlightenment as seen in the above historical descriptions. This is similar to the modern tai chi practitioners' emphasis on its martial arts aspect without knowing the original Daoist' practice of tai chi is to prepare the body and the mind complex for the development of the sudden enlightenment of Shen ming. For the invention of tai chi the legendary Daoist, Zhang Sanfend, shown in the following picture is similar to Bodhidharma's role in the development of Chan Buddhism.

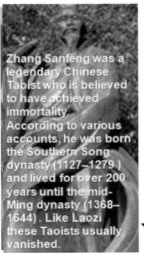

Zhang Sanfeng was a legendary Chinese Taoist who is believed to have achieved immortality. According to various accounts, he was born the Southern Song dynasty (1127–1279) and lived for over 200 years until the mid-Ming dynasty (1368–1644). Like Laozi these Taoists usually vanished.

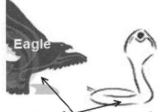

Eagle

A coiled up snake defeated its deadly predator, the eagle triggered the invention of tai chi by the Taoist, Zhang Sanfeng.

The illustrations in the picture have been enlarged in the following picture:

Zhang Sanfeng was a legendary Chinese Taoist who is believed to have achieved immortality. According to various accounts, he was born the Southern Song dynasty (1127–1279) and lived for over 200 years until the mid-Ming dynasty (1368–1644). Like Laozi these Taoists usually vanished.

This legendary origin of tai chi by a Daoist has not been confirmed by historical records but the development of tai chi from the original purpose of super mental enrichment, called Shen ming to the later commercialization of its practice into a form of martial arts or exercise that creates monetary opportunities is similar to the same development of the birth of Chan Buddhism for spiritual enlightenment at Shaolin Temple and its later mutation into a school of martial arts , headed by the current abbot of the Shaolin Temple，Shi Yongxin 释永信, who has been notoriously nick named as the "CEO Monk" . To read the long list of criticisms of his commercialization of Shaolin Temple please Google, "Shi Yongxin 释永信". You can use his Chinese name or the pinyin, Shi Yongxin.

2/The following breathing practice with a set of detailed instructions shows us one way of reaching 神明 (Shén míng, enlightenment) in the opening quotation of this article, "<u>由著熟而漸悟懂勁，由懂勁而階及神明，然非用力之久，不能豁然貫通焉</u>....。".

In Chan 禪 Buddhism and in Tibetan Buddhism if one can practice the Nine Sessions Buddhist wind breathing method, 九節佛風 Jiǔ jié fú fēng to a sophisticated level the practitioner can reach a breathing mode called, Bǎo píng qì 寶瓶氣. (Its instructional video with English subtitles of this breathing practice is available on YouTube: https://www.youtube.com/watch?v=Za0wxuF4jlg

南老师示范九节佛风及宝瓶气 (Eng Sub) ,uploaded by TransparentSeed)

From this Bǎo píng qì state, which is equivalent to the state of "Dong jin" in tai chi the practitioner could get enlightenment if he or she practices Buddhism or Immortality if he or she practices Daoism.

The most basic requirement in reaching Bǎo píng qì 寶瓶氣 is to be able to hold your breath for 72 seconds, according to Master Nan, at 19 minute of the above movie.

These religious goals are examples of the state, called 神明 Shén míng.

《太極拳論》·山右　王宗岳
https://zh.wikipedia.org/wiki/太極拳論:

"虛領頂勁，氣沉丹田。不偏不倚，忽隱忽現。左重則左虛，右重則右杳。仰之則彌高，俯之則彌深。進之則愈長，退之則愈促。一羽不能加，蠅蟲不能落。人不知我，我獨知人，英雄所向無敵，蓋皆由此而及也。

斯技旁門甚多，雖勢有區別，概不外乎壯欺弱、慢讓快耳。有力打無力，手慢讓手快，是皆先天自然之能，非關學力而有為也。察「四兩撥千斤」之句，顯非力勝；觀耄耋能禦眾之形，快何能為？

立如平準，活似車輪，偏沉則隨，雙重則滯。每見數年純功，不能運化者，率皆自為人制，雙重之病未悟耳。欲避此病，須知陰陽。粘即是走，走即是粘，陰不離陽，陽不離陰，陰陽相濟，方為懂勁。懂勁後，愈練愈精，默識揣摩，漸至從心所欲。本是「捨己從人」，多誤「捨近求遠」，所謂「差之毫厘，謬之千里」，學者不可不詳辨焉，是為論。"

註云 **A footnote of the above tai chi classics has been added by Jiang Fa** 蔣發：「此論句句切要在心，並無一字陪襯，非有夙慧（**sù huì**）之人，未能悟也，先師不肯妄傳，非獨擇人，亦恐枉費工夫耳」。

蔣發 **Jiang Fa was born in 1574 during the Ming Dynasty of China** 明萬曆二年.

My translation of his footnote:

"My teacher was very selective when teaching tai chi. He said tai chi was hard to teach to students who did not have 夙慧（**sù huì**）**."**

According to Buddhist beliefs 夙慧（**sù huì**）**is a form of innate intelligence formed from one's former life's merits and good deeds.**

*王宗岳 *Zongyue* Wang's 《*太極拳論 Tai Chi quán lùn*》, "… 太極者，無極而生，動靜之機，陰陽之母也。動之則分，靜之則合*。…"

The following anecdotes recorded in a book, 《拳意述真》 written by MasterSun Lutang, the founder of Sun style tai chi are concrete manifestations of Shen ming, the miraculous ability of practitioners, who have reached this Enlightenment state. The way how Master Sun died is also an illustration of the Daoist kind of Enlightenment, which is a form of Shen ming:

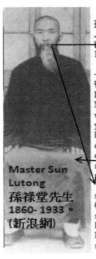

【無疾而終·含笑面逝·震驚當世】

孫錄堂晚年隱居鄉間，預言自己逝世之日，不食者兩旬(應類似修道人之靜坐閉關之禁食)，每日練拳書字無間，臨終時，面朝東南奇袈西北，端坐椅上，囑家人勿哭並曰「吾視死生如遊戲耳。」於1933年清晨六時五分含笑面逝；當世震驚，《申報》《民國日報》《大公報》《益世報》《世界日報》等重要報刊均作報導並給孫之一生高度評價；南京、上海、杭州、北平、天津各武術團體紛紛舉行公祭追悼。[Wikipedia]

English translation of the above illustrations:
Master Sun stunned the world when he ended his life in a Daoist's way of self-administered euthanasia to enter immortality. In his late years, Master Sun Lutang was living in retirement in the countryside; he predicted the day of his death and practiced 辟穀 Bi Gu for two days (for an enlightened Daoist, Bi Gu means to stop eating before his or her spirit leaves the physical body.) When the time came he sat on a chair in a Confucian manner, facing southwest with his back to the northwest and told the family members not to cry and said to them, "I regard death only as a game." At 6:05 AM in 1933 he died with a smile. The major Chinese newspapers and magazines such as the 《申報》《民國日報》《大公報》《益世報》《世界日報》 reported his special way to die like an enlightened Daoist. All the editorials spoke highly of him. In major cities like Nanjing, Shanghai, Hangzhou, Beijing, and Tianjin many martial arts groups held public memorial services for Master Sun.

Master Sun Lutong
孫祿堂先生
1860- 1933 。
(新浪網)

https://zh.wikipedia.org/wiki/孫祿堂

English translation of the above illustrations of Master Sun Lutang can be read below:

Master Sun stunned the world when he ended his life in a Daoist's way of self-administered euthanasia to enter another state of his life, immortality. In his late years, Master Sun Lutang was living in retirement in the countryside; he predicted the day of his death and practiced 辟穀 Bi Gu for two days (for an enlightened Daoist, Bi Gu means eating only a small amount of raw food and eventually to stop eating before his or her spirit leaves the physical body.) When the time came he sat on a chair in a Confucian manner, facing southwest with his back to the northwest and told the family members not to cry and said to them, "I regard death only as a game." At 6:05 AM in 1933 he died with a smile. The major Chinese newspapers and magazines such as the 《申報》《民國日報》《大公報》《益世報》《世界日報》 reported his special way to die like an enlightened Daoist. All the editorials spoke highly of him. In major cities like Nanjing, Shanghai, Hangzhou, Beijing, and Tianjin many martial arts groups held public memorial services for Master Sun.

This is the original Chinese publication in Wikipedia:

【無疾而終·含笑而逝·震驚當世】

孫錄堂晚年隱居鄉間，預言自己逝世之日，不食者兩旬(應類似修道人之靜坐閉關之禁食)，每日練拳書字無間，臨終時，面朝東南背靠西北，端坐椅上，囑家人勿哀哭並曰:「吾視死生如遊戲耳。」[來源請求]於1933年清晨六時五分含笑而逝；當世震驚，《申報》《民國日報》《大公報》《益世報》《世界日報》等重要報刊均作報導並給孫之一生高度評價；南京、上海、杭州、北平、天津各武術團體紛紛舉行公祭追悼。(Translated from https://zh.wikipedia.org/wiki/孫祿堂)

李洛能 Master Li Luoneng's legendary kung fu can be estimated from an incident, reported by Sun Lutang one of his inner circle students in Sun's book 《拳意述真》, "…本境有某甲，武進士也，體力逾常人，兼善拳術，與先生素相善，而於先生之武術，則竊有不服，每蓄意相較，輒以相善之故，難於啟齒。一日會談一室，言笑一如平常，初不料某甲之蓄意相試，毫無防備之意，而某甲於先生行動時，乘其不意，竊於身後即捉住先生，用力舉起。及一伸手，而身體已騰空斜上，頭顱觸入頂棚之內，復行落下，兩足仍直立於地，未嘗傾跌。以邪術疑先生，先生告之曰：是非邪術也，蓋拳術上乘神化之功，有不見不聞之知覺，故神妙若此，非汝之所知也。時人遂稱先生曰：神拳李能然。年八十餘歲，端坐椅上，一笑而逝。

Master Li Luoneng's legendary kung fu was mentioned bySun Lutang in his book in the website, 拳意述真: 拳意述真- 中国哲学书电子化计划

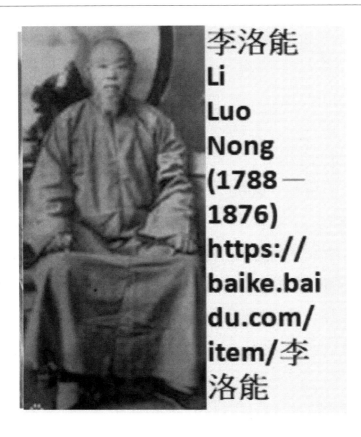

李洛能 Li Luo Nong (1788－1876) https://baike.baidu.com/item/李洛能

Source of the above picture:

https://baike.baidu.com/item/李洛能

172　拳術至練虛合道，是將真意化到至虛至無之境，不動之時，內中寂然，空虛無一動其心，至於忽然有不測之事，雖不見不聞而能覺而避之。中庸云：「至誠之道可以前知」，是此意也。能到至誠之道者，三派拳術中，餘知有四人而已。形意拳李洛能先生，八卦拳董海川先生，太極拳楊露禪先生，武禹襄先生。四位先生皆有不見不聞之知覺。其餘諸先生，皆是見聞之知覺而已。如外不有測之事，只要眼見耳聞，無論來者如何疾快，俱能躲閃。因其功夫入於虛境而未到於至虛，不能有不見不聞之知覺也。其練他派拳術者，亦常聞有此境界，未能詳其姓氏，故未錄之。

The following is the English translation of the above quotations: Among Master Neng-ran Li's close friends there was an exceptionally strong martial artist, who had achieved the honour in the State martial artist examination as one of the group of distinguished martial artists. He wanted to compare his kung fu with Master Li's but he did not want to challenge him in an open tournament. One day they were engaged in conversation as usual. This man held and lifted Master Li up forcefully from behind by surprise. He could feel that Master Li had been lifted up so high that his head was touching the ceiling.

However, Master Li's feet were still standing on the ground. At first that man thought Master Li was using a magic trick. Master Li explained that his martial art practice was similar to the Daoist practice and in the advance stage of this religious practice 神通 Sheng Tong, a miraculous protection would automatically manifest itself to protect the practitioner. Any martial artist with the protection of this form of miracle is invincible. Because of his advanced martial art accomplishment, he was nicknamed God's punch Master Li. When he was eighty-one he passed away like an enlightened Daoist, , sitting in a chair in a Confucian manner; smiled and died. MasterSun Lutang died in the same manner.

172 In the most advanced state martial arts is similar to Laozi's Daoism it is united to the universal Dao and therefore has the same miraculous quality to predict when is going to happen from some early signs. According to the Confucian Doctrine of the Mean, called 中庸, one of the Four Books in the Confucian Ethics, this manifestation of the advanced form of martial arts is referred to as, "至誠之道,可以前知…". It means that at the sophisticated level of one's religious or ethical belief one possesses the premonition to sense what is going to happen from forthcoming signs that usually occur before an abrupt change of event.   I (Sun) know that there are at least four martial arts masters, who possess this miraculous ability, Master 李洛能 Li Luoneng of Xingyiquan, Master 董海川 Dong Haichuan of Baqua quan, Master 楊露禪 Yang Luchen of Taijiquan,

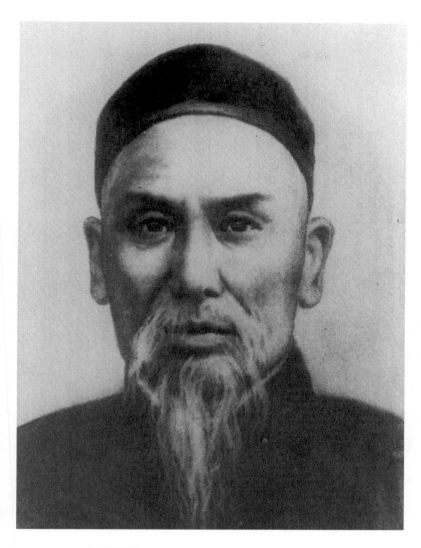

(Master 楊露禪 Yang Luchen of Taijiquan)

and Master 武禹襄

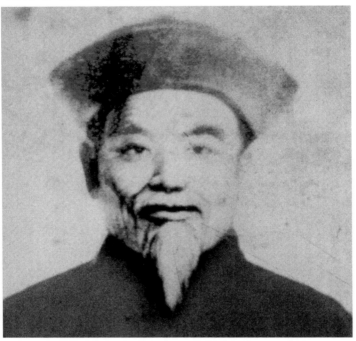
of

Taijiquan. There are quite a few masters possessing
this ability. However, since I do not know their names
and cannot mention them.

According to Sun Lutang 《拳意述真》35

董海川(1797－1882): 董海川先生,順天文安縣,朱家塢人,喜習武術,嘗涉跡江皖間,遇異人傳授,居三年,拳術劍術及各器械,無不造其極,歸後入睿王府當差,人多知其有奇技異能,投為門下受教者絡繹不絕,所教拳術,稱為八卦,其式形,皆是河圖洛書之數,其道體,俱是先生後天之理,其用法,乃八八六十四卦之變化而無窮,一部易理,先生方寸之間,體之無遺,是以先生行止坐臥,動作之際,其變化之神妙,非常人所能測也,居嘗跏趺靜坐,值夏日大雨牆忽傾倒,時先生跌坐於坑貼近此牆,先生並未開目,弟子在側者,見牆倒之時,急注視先生忽不見,而先生已跌坐,於他處之椅上,身上未著點塵,先生又嘗晝寢,時值深秋,弟子以被覆之,輕輕覆於先生身,不意被覆於床,存者僅床與被,而先生不見矣,驚而返顧,則先生端坐於臨廳之一椅,謂其人曰,何不言耶,使我一驚,蓋先生之靈機至是,已臻不見不聞,即可知覺之境,故臨不測之,其變化之神妙,有如此者,中庸云,至誠之道,可以前知,即此義也,

年八十餘歲,端坐而逝,弟子尹福,程廷華等,

葬於東直門外,榛椒樹東北,紅橋大道旁,諸門弟子建碑,以志其行為。

https://ctext.org/wiki.pl?if=en&chapter=en&chapter=909446&searchu=董海川

Dong Haichuan (1797-1882): Master Dong Haichuan resided for three years with a gifted kung fu master, from whom he learned his martial arts. Then he worked for one of the royal members of the Qing Dynasty. In spite of his low status as a servant many people admired his skills in kung fu and he had many followers. His kung fu was founded on the numerous combinations of the 64 trigrams of I Jing and Daoism. He seemed to possess the miraculous power as an enlightened Daoist to predict things that were going to happen. At one time he was meditating in a double lotus sitting style on a bed right besides a wall. It was raining very hard. The wall collapsed. But it did not hurt him because he had moved to a safe spot and his students did not know how he did this move when he was in a meditative state with his eyes closed with his posture locked in a double lotus sitting style. His move was so quick that his clothes did not even catch a bit of the mud or dust from the collapsed wall.

At another time his student was trying to cover him with a blanket, but he disappeared when the blanket was put on. Then his student saw him sitting at the other end of the room and he was asking his student why he didn't let him know before putting on a blanket on him. According to the Confucian Doctrine of the Mean, called 中庸, one of the Four Books in the Confucian Ethics, this manifestation of the advanced form of martial arts is referred to as, "至誠之道,可以前知,即此義也". It means that at the sophisticated level of one's religious or ethical belief one possesses the premonition to sense what is going to happen from forthcoming signs that usually occur before an abrupt change of event. This could account for Master Dong's aforementioned miraculous ability. Master Dong died in a self-administered euthanasia way when he was in his eighties. He sat on a chair in a Confucian sitting manner and died peacefully. His disciples 尹福 Yin Fu and ,程廷華 Cheng Tinghua buried him in 東直門 Dongzhimen, northeast of a hazelnut tree, next to 紅橋大道 Hongqiao Avenue; a tablet was erected to honour Master Dong's achievements.

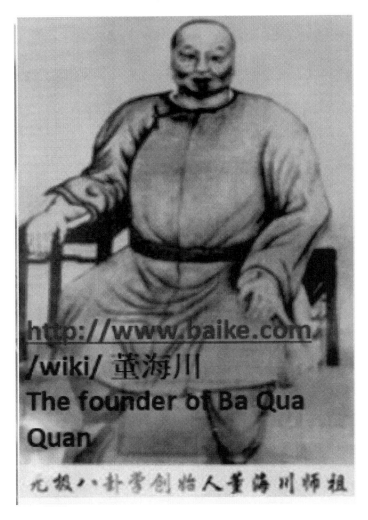

http://www.baike.com
/wiki/ 董海川
The founder of Ba Qua
Quan

3/Between 著熟(Zhe shú, meaning to have known the movements by heart)**and** 懂勁(Dong jin) Yang Chengfu added 鬆開 "Song kai" :

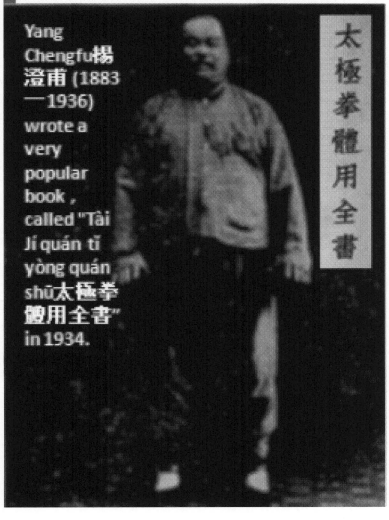

"鬆開 Song kai" was one of the key principles in Tai Chi that was heavily emphasized by Master Chengfu Yang

Yang Chengfu楊澄甫 (1883—1936) wrote a very popular book, called "Tài Jí quán tǐ yòng quán shū太極拳體用全書" in 1934.

太極拳體用全書

One of the signs of "Song kai" is Ding Tou Xuan 頂頭懸 of the CranioSacral postural reflex in Tai Chi because when you feel Ding Tou Xuan, meaning that the head is as light as if it was hanging in the air the shoulder and neck have to be in a "Song kai" state as shown in the above picture.

To a large extent Ding Tou Xuan 頂 頭 懸 is formed from the suction of the throat Dantian of the pharyngeal region of the lower neck.

The Pharyngeal cavity is where the throat Dantian functions.

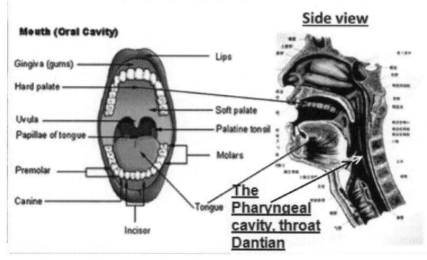

have uploaded a few movies on YouTube regarding Dantian singing and how to exercise the lingual and pharyngeal muscles in a tai chi way with adhesion so that the singing has the unique Chinese opera singing characteristics of 韻味 Yùnwèi, the lingering charm of various forms of art like singing or painting. For more details please watch the following movies on YouTube:

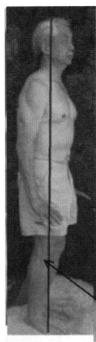

韻味 Yùnwèi the latent and lingering charm of martial art can be felt even in the pictures of 椿功 Zhuāng gōng

The beginning pose of tai chi as a form of 椿功 Zhuāng gōng demonstrated by Dr. George Ho

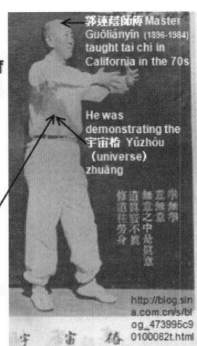

郭連蔭師傅 Master Guōliányīn (1896-1984) taught tai chi in California in the 70s

He was demonstrating the 宇宙椿 Yǔzhòu (universe) zhuāng

學無意意無意意之中是直意
道修身道化勞身
無意之中是直意

http://blog.sina.com.cn/s/blog_473995c90100082t.html

宇 宙 椿

https://www.youtube.com/watch?v=ov5ObN82mFowei Dantian 丹田 manifestation, 韻味 Yùnwèi a unique characteristic in Chinese art including martial arts

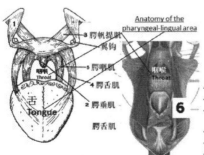

Anatomy of the pharyngeal-lingual area

The Pharyngeal Muscles
- 1/The leveator veli palatini muscle 顎帆提肌
- 2/uvulae 懸雍垂肌
- 3/the tensor veli palatini 顎帆張肌 The soft palate 軟顎
- 4/palatoglossus 顎舌肌
- 5/palatopharyngeus 顎咽肌
- 6/The salpingopharyngeus muscle 耳咽管咽肌

Chiropractic doctor: Dr. George K.W. Ho of Vancouver
For my original movies with their comments please go to my YouTube channel, Dr. George Ho.
溫哥華：何錦榮 (Kam Wing) 脊醫 香港政府註冊
My logo

https://www.youtube.com/watch?v=fe-PoZkQKYI

The illustrations in the picture have been enlarged in the following picture:

The Pharyngeal Muscles

- 1/The levetor veli palatini muscle颚帆提肌
- 2/uvulae 懸雍垂肌
- 3/the tensor veli palatini 顎帆張肌
  The soft palate軟顎
- 4/palatoglossus顎舌肌
- 5/palatopharyngeus顎咽肌
- 6/The salpingopharyngeus muscle耳咽管咽肌

(1)Tai chi breathing cultivated by Dantian singing as a form of throat and tongue tai chi

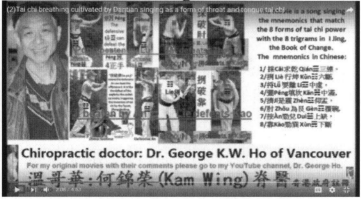

https://www.youtube.com/watch?v=5i0dN9zryQ8

The illustrations in the picture have been enlarged in the following picture:

ngue tai chi/le is a song singing the mnemonics that match the 8 forms of tai chi power with the 8 trigrams in I Jing, the Book of Change.
The mnemonics in Chinese:

1/ 採Cǎi求乾 Qián☰ 三連，
2/ 挒Liè 行坤 Kūn☷ 六斷，
3/ 捋Lǚ 要離 Lí☲ 中虛，
4/ 掤Péng填坎 Kǎn☵ 中滿，
5/ 擠㪉足震 Zhèn☳ 仰盂，
6/ 肘Zhǒu 為艮 Gèn☶ 覆碗，
7/ 按Àn勁兌 Duì☱ 上缺，
8/ 靠Kào勁巽 Xùn☴ 下斷

enlarged in the following picture:

The Importance of the CranioSacral postural reflex in Tai Chi by
Dr. George Ho, B.Soc. Sc.,M.A.,D.C.

"鬆開 Song kai" was one of the key principles in Tai Chi that was heavily emphasized by Master Chengfu Yang 楊澄甫 (1883-1936), the 3rd generation representative of Yang style Tai Chi. He emphasized that in practice as well as in real combats the whole body has to be in a "鬆開 Song kai" state. Otherwise one will be forced into the defensive and reactive status all the time.

One of his students, Master Man-ching Cheng 鄭 曼青 (1902－1975）was the 4th generation representative of Yang style Tai Chi. He said it took him 50 years to really experience what his teacher, Master Chengfu Yang 楊澄甫 meant by " 鬆開 Song kai" , translated by鄭Cheng's team of students as a state of "relaxation". 曼青亲訴紀述：「澄師每日必重言十餘次，要鬆要鬆；要鬆淨，要全身鬆開，反之則日不鬆，不鬆，不鬆就是挨打的架子，」(鄭)

One of Master Man-ching Cheng students, Mr. Benjamin Lo (Luóbǎngzhēn羅邦楨, 1925-) of San Francisco was asked in an interview in 2001 regarding the main principles of Tai Chi. He maintained that "relaxation" was the most important one and when he was asked how to become relaxed he said doing the Tai Chi forms was the only way he knew. He said doing the forms would lead to the posture to acquire this elusive state of "relaxation".

(2) Tai chi breathing cultivated by Dantian singing as a form of throat and tongue tai chi

For a better singing demonstration of my opera singing that has 韻味 Yùnwèi please watch the following movie in Chinesehttps://www.youtube.com/watch?v=UO0TvixMP28&list=PL9RRMUY60ixTdZpWGySNpmYtCPSmegRpk
https://www.youtube.com/watch?v=Mv0i91uVDWg
唱好歌就是呼吸的藝術, Cantonese opera,(1)夜半歌聲 by Dr. George Ho All copyrights reserved

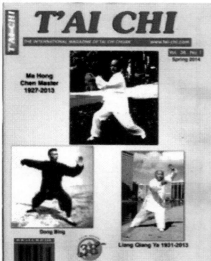

T'AI CHI

THE INTERNATIONAL MAGAZINE OF T'AI CHI CH'UAN   www.tai-chi.com

Vol. 38, No. 1
Spring 2014

Ma Hong
Chen Master
1927-2013

Dong Bing

Liang Qiang Ya 1931-2013

My article in the 2014 Spring issue of T'ai Chi Magazine

The Importance of the CranioSacral postural reflex in Tai Chi by Dr. George Ho, B.Soc. Sc.,M.A.,D.C.

"超鬆 Song kai" was one of the key principles in Tai Chi that was heavily emphasized by Master Chengfu Yang 楊澄甫 (1883-1936), the 3rd generation representative of Yang style Tai Chi. He emphasized that in practice as well as in real combats the whole body has to be in a "超鬆 Song kai" state. Otherwise one will be forced into the defensive and reactive status all the time.

One of his students, Master Man-ching Cheng 鄭 曼青 (1902—1975) was the 4th generation representative of Yang style Tai Chi. He said it took him 50 years to really experience what his teacher, Master Chengfu Yang 楊澄甫 meant by " 超鬆 Song kai" , translated by鄭Cheng's team of students as a state of "relaxation". 曼青亲折秘述： 「澄所每日必重言十餘次，要鬆要鬆：要鬆淨，要全身鬆開，反之則曰不鬆，不鬆，不鬆就是挨打的架子。」(郑)

One of Master Man-ching Cheng students, Mr. Benjamin Lo (Luóbāngzhēn羅邦楨, 1925-) of San Francisco was asked in an interview in 2001 regarding the main principles of Tai Chi. He maintained that "relaxation" was the most important one and when he was asked how to become relaxed he said doing the Tai Chi forms was the only way he knew. He said doing the forms would lead to the posture to acquire this elusive state of "relaxation".

6

For a detailed discussion of "Song kai" please read my article, The CranioSacral postural reflex in Tai Chi Part 2, introduced by my YouTube movie:

https://www.youtube.com/watch?v=OJVbymIYjQM

"Beyond Relaxation" in tai chi and therapeutic seminars using tai chi power

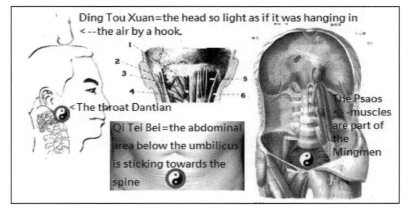

The illustrations in the picture have been enlarged in the following picture:

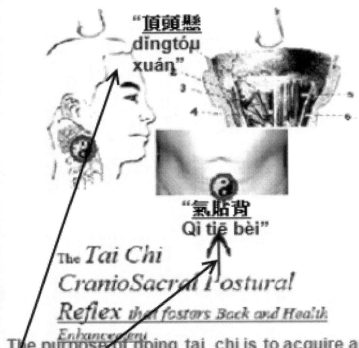

"頂頭懸
dǐngtóμ
xuáŋ"

"氣貼背
Qi tiē bèi"

The *Tai Chi CranioSacral Postural Reflex that fosters Back and Health Enhancement.*

The purpose of doing tai chi is to acquire an unique postural reflex that makes you feel the head as light as if it was hanging in the air and the abdominal part below the umbilicus sticks towards the spine.

This new concept, "the CranioSacral Postural reflex of tai chi" was created by Dr. George Ho, D.C. who owns its copyrights.

4/When your body is in a "Song kai" state you can efficiently "store up power like a bow being drawn and release it like a heavily loaded arrow 蓄勁如張弓，發勁如放箭", according to Yǔxiāng Wǔ's (1812-1880) 武禹襄《*太極拳解 Tàijí quán jiě*》

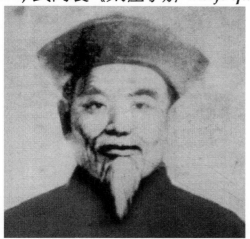

A picture of Wǔyǔxiāng 武禹襄

Dǒng 懂 in Chinese literally means to know and jìn 勁 means strength. Dǒng jìn can be better visualized in the aforementioned concrete expressions of "storing up power like a bow being drawn and release it like a heavily loaded arrow 蓄勁如張弓，發勁如放箭", according to Yǔxiāng Wǔ's (1812-1880) 武禹襄. This is the goal of your practice in the 著熟 (Zhe shú) state, which is the reason why the movements are done slowly so that you can practice "loading the body with power" like a drawn bow and releasing the power like an arrow. When the 著熟 (Zhe shú) is sophisticated "Song kai" will occur naturally.

5/ After reaching this state of dǒng jìn one's Tai Chi kung fu can improve qualitatively by the continuous practice of the complementary cooperative actions of the yin and the yang. The more one practices the better the Tai Chi dǒng jìn kung fu will become. The original text of the above translation is as followed, "陰 陽 相濟方為懂勁。懂勁後。愈練愈精。" (陰 =yin, 陽=yang, 相濟= complementing each other, 方為懂勁。懂勁後 =after the acquisition of dong jin。愈練愈精 =continuous improvement。

The significance of the above quote is as followed:

"蓄勁 Xù jìn 如張弓(a drawn bow)，發勁 fā jìn 如放箭(a shooting arrow)."

蓄勁 Xù jìn represents the 陰 =yin, the power storing state like a bow in the process of being drawn and 發勁 fā jìn represents the 陽=yang state like a fully drawn bow shooting an arrow. When they can 相濟= complement each other, you have reached the 方為懂勁 (dong jin) state. This is the goal and the principle when you practice your tai chi movements.

The above principle actually applies to any sports or skill. It is called practice makes perfect.

6/ The most significant mind body enhancement transformation is the state after "懂勁 dong jin", called the 神明 Shén míng state.

由 from"懂勁 dong jin"而 Jiē jí 階及(step onto)神明 Shén míng，然非用力之久(after a prolonged period of diligent practice)，不能(豁然 Huò rán= Suddenly)(貫通 Guàn Tōng=breakthrough)。

My paraphrased translation of the above quote:

After a prolonged practice the new mind body movement of tai chi with the CranioSacral postural reflex and the eight forms of tai chi power you could experience a sudden mind body sublimation similar to the acquisition of the balance reflex to ride a bicycle.

7/ I would like to add that many enlightened scholars like 南懷瑾 Nán Huái jǐn went one step further with this tai chi Dong jin level to practice Chan meditation and reached their coveted enlightenment, called 頓悟 (Dùn wù) in Chan Buddhism.

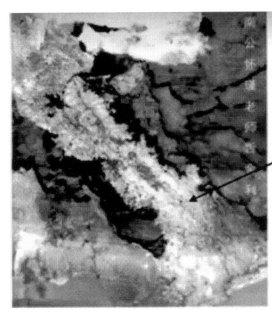

After cremation Master Nan's tongue remained intact and was covered with lotus-shaped holy relics.

南師懷瑾荼毘 (tú pí)後，舌頭完整，上面佈滿蓮花狀舍利子！

The illustrations in the picture have been enlarged in the following picture:

After cremation Master Nan's tongue remained intact and was covered with lotus-shaped holy relics.

南師懷瑾荼毘
(tú pí)後，舌頭
完整，上面佈滿
蓮花狀舍利子！

Nan Huai-Chin 南懷瑾, (1918 – 2012) was a spiritual teacher of contemporary China. He was the most eminent disciple of the lay Chan Buddhist teacher Yuan Huan xian, and received confirmation of his enlightenment by various masters of the Buddhist traditions. He was considered by many to be the major force in the revival of Chinese Buddhism.

Nán Huái jǐn practiced Yang style tai chi when he was in his middle age but in his old age he only practiced Chan meditation.

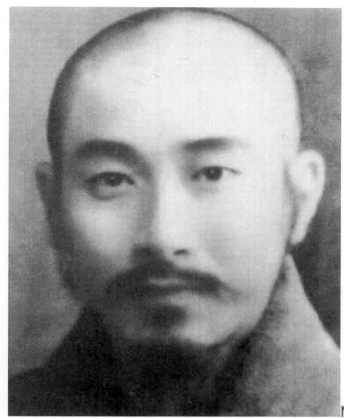

Nan Huai-Chin

in 1945, after descending **Mount Emei** from his hermitage.

https://en.wikipedia.org/wiki/Nan_Huai-Chin)

Master Nan talked about a concrete example of the 神明 Shén míng state : "密宗強調修氣，在修氣以前，這些道理先要懂得。修氣修到不呼不吸，呼吸停止，密宗叫"寶瓶氣"，瑜珈術稱"瓶氣"。人像寶瓶一樣，在定境要來時，氣充滿了，呼吸停掉，肚子回收進去，身子自然直了，端端正正，定住了，這時舒服得很，叫你下坐都不干。

不呼也不吸，並不是真正沒有呼吸，只是很細微而已。此時雜念沒有了，過了很久，好像有一點吸進來；很久以後，又有一點呼出去，到這個境界就要修脈了。這是唐代以後密宗的說法。

知息冷知息暖，就是在修脈的境界，但並不是在鼻端知息冷暖，而是在身體內部，此時，在身體內部知道哪裡發暖，哪裡發冷，這就是後世密宗所說的脈，差不多相對於神經反應。每個細胞的感覺，哪裡走得通，哪裡走不通，都清楚。事實上，脈就是息的更進一步。

打坐為什麼腿麻？因為腿的脈不通，下部的脈都沒有通。最難通的是臀部，我們坐到後來不想坐了，有兩個原因，一個是心，一個是身。通常我們不想坐了，是不是心不想坐？不是的，大部分是因為氣到臀部沉不下去了，此時氣會影響心理。凡夫的心不能轉物，唯物思想家認為，人的思想受物理影響，並沒有錯，只是這個說法只適應在凡夫的境界上。氣也是物，所以我們坐到某一階段時，因為氣到臀部沉不下去了，無形中腦神經緊張起來，心裡就坐不住了，只好下座。如果氣從臀部通到大腿、膝蓋，一節節通下來，要經歷過痛、癢、麻、脹、冷、熱、甚至兩腿發爛，最後等氣一走通，忽然就好了。古代修行人，修持精神很可佩，氣把身體內部的髒東西逼出來，逼到身體都爛了，他們也能把色陰看空，毫不在乎。現在的人有福氣了，只要吃消炎藥，打消炎針就行。

待氣到了足心，才能談得到三脈七輪。氣脈打通了，準可得定，得哪種定？定有百千三昧，每種不同，而我們卻以為只有一個"禪"。所以說，為何禪宗以後更無禪，禪是真誤了不少人。

真正把中脈打通了以後，一坐一定，閉著眼，滿天星斗看得清清楚楚，密宗所講的是真事。那個情景就像太空船進入太空的境界一樣，這就是宇宙的奧秘，生命的奧秘。上次太空船進入太空的整個過程，每一秒我都留意其變化，注意宇宙間的法則，是否和人體是一樣的，結果發現完全一樣。由此更證明，佛法顯密所說的修持經驗，一點都沒有錯，錯在我們自己不用功，沒有修證到。 ---《如何修證佛法*》

*南懷瑾(1996). *如何修證佛法*.臺北.老古文化事業股份有限公司.p.163-165

My paraphrased translation of the above talk:
Tibetan Buddhism emphasises the cultivation of Qi.
One of the goals of this cultivation is to reach a mental physical state, called 寶瓶氣, Bao ping qi, when the prolonged breathing practice of a form of pranayama, called Nine Sessions Buddhist Wind Breathing,九節佛風 Jiǔ jié fú fēng

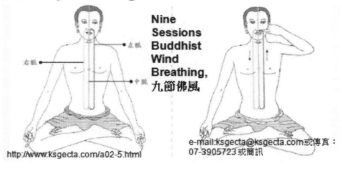

Nine Sessions Buddhist Wind Breathing, 九節佛風

左脈
右脈
中脈

http://www.ksgecta.com/a02-5.html

e-mail:ksgecta@ksgecta.com或傳真：
07-3905723 或簡訊

has transformed the body's quality into a state in which minimal breathing is needed to sustain the survival of the practitioner who has entered the mental physical condition, called 定 Dìng. For 禪 Chán practitioners it is called 禪定 Chán ding.

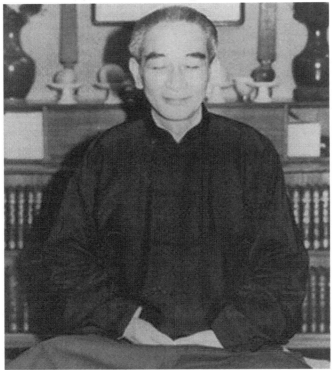

南怀瑾 http://bodhi.takungpao.com/sspt/sraddha/2016-01/3264206.html

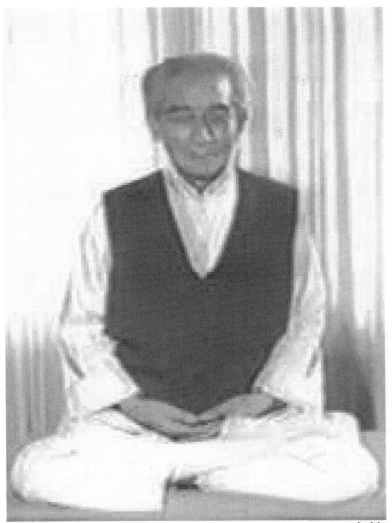

http://luzifur.pixnet.net/blog/post/9934379-南懷瑾的坐姿示範圖

It is in this state of Ding that qi refines the dormant meridians, especially the Central Meridian, housed by the spine that includes the skull and the sacrum.

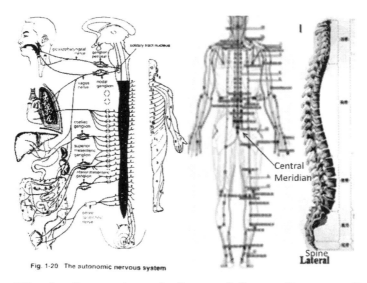

Fig. 1-20 The autonomic nervous system

The body posture is formed from the way the practitioner practices.

←Double lotus sitting like Buddha is not the only way.

Other postures include **side lying ones and standing ones;** the middle picture shows a standing Lohan 羅漢. Meditative walking is also an option.

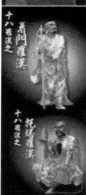

Practicing meditation in different postures to obtain enlightenment have been exemplified by several hundreds of Lohan 羅漢, perfected persons who had attained nirvana.

Even nowadays in India there are people practicing meditation in one posture for decades without any postural changes.

←The bottom picture show a Lohan who held a pagoda in his hand all the time to commemorate Buddha.

The illustrations in the picture have been enlarged in the following picture:

← **Double lotus sitting** like Buddha is not the only way.

Other postures include **side lying ones and standing ones;** the middle picture shows a standing Lohan 羅漢. Meditative walking is also an option.

Practicing meditation in different postures to obtain enlightenment have been exemplified by several hundreds of Lohan 羅漢, perfected persons who had attained nirvana.

Even nowadays in India there are people practicing meditation in one posture for decades without any postural changes.

← The bottom picture show a Lohan who held a pagoda in his hand all the time to commemorate Buddha.

8/Any posture as exemplified by all the Buddhist statues is possible for this state to emerge as long as it has the CranioSacral postural reflex of tai chi, the weight-less feeling of the head, called Ding Tou Xuan 頂頭懸 and an adhesive feeling of the abdominal part below the umbilicus, called Qi Tie Bai 氣貼背 when the practitioner feels that the aforementioned anatomical part is sticking towards the spine.

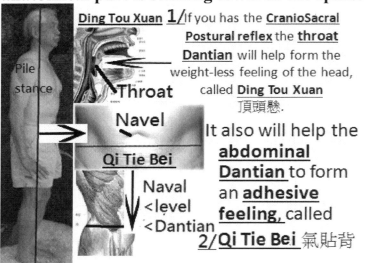

Ding Tou Xuan 1/If you has the CranioSacral Postural reflex the throat Dantian will help form the weight-less feeling of the head, called Ding Tou Xuan 頂頭懸.

It also will help the **abdominal Dantian** to form an **adhesive feeling,** called 2/**Qi Tie Bei** 氣貼背

Pile stance

Throat

Navel

Qi Tie Bei

Naval
<level
<Dantian

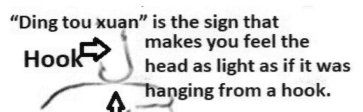

"Ding tou xuan" is the sign that makes you feel the head as light as if it was hanging from a hook.

Hook

"Ding tou xuan"

The throat Dantian

Dīng tóu xuán

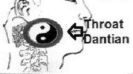

"頂頭懸 Dǐng tóu xuán" meaning, the head feels as light as if it was floating in the air, hanging by a hook.

Throat Dantian

Qi tiē bèi

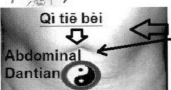

Abdominal Dantian

"氣貼背 Qì tiē bèi" means the Abdominal Dantian, abdominal part below the umbilicus seems to adhere toward the spine and the adhesion intensifies with the tai chi movements.

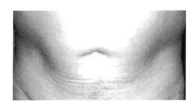

This stomach has acquired the 'Qi sticking towards the spine', the source of tai chi power

When this Ding 定 mental physical state has been cultivated the accumulating qi will refine the meridians of the body from head to toes. From experiences practitioners said that the gluteal buttock region is the most difficult anatomical part for the qi to penetrate. When the meridian refinement is complete from the 百會穴 Bǎi huì xué acupuncture point to the 湧泉穴 yǒng quán xué acupunctures point

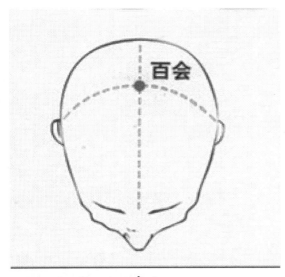

百會穴 Bǎi huì xué

acupuncture point

The left foot 湧泉穴 (yǒng quán xué) is Earth Branch 3 寅 yin and the right 湧泉穴 is Earth Branch 12 亥 hai.

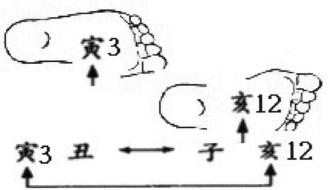

of the soles of the feet it is a state very close if not into the state of Enlightenment.

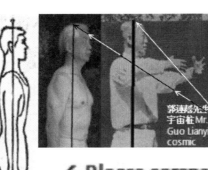

郭连荫先生
宇宙桩 Mr.
Guo Lianyin
cosmic

← Please compare the generally accepted normal posture on the far left with the basic tai chi stance posture of Dr. Ho in the middle. The former's central line of gravity passes from the top of the head, the 百會 穴 Bǎi huì acupuncture point to the rear foot whereas the ... he tai ...ore the 湧 ...é ...at the up the ...eract al pull; ...rtant art for ...oting.

← Please compare the generally accepted normal posture on the far left with the basic tai chi stance posture of Dr. Ho in the middle. The former's central line of gravity passes from the top of the head, the 百會 穴 Bǎi huì acupuncture point to the rear foot whereas the comparative line in the tai chi stance passes more towards the forefoot, the 湧 泉穴 yǒng quán xué acupuncture point so that the feet can actively link up the whole body to counteract the earth's gravitational pull; this is the most important practice of all martial art for real kung fu, called rooting.

The illustrations in the picture have been enlarged in the following picture:

The preparatory pose of tai chi, shown above is one example of the postural requirements to enter the mental physical state of Ding 定.

9/After reaching this 神明 Shén míng state the extremely hard to reach 頓悟(Dùn wù) state in Chan 禪 Buddhism could occur when the time comes.

After one has acquired 懂勁 (Dong jin) but do not step (階及) into the further refinement to reach the 神明 Shén míng then one has missed the most important goal of practicing tai chi, the martial arts aspect of which is the least important according to the tai chi founder, 張三丰 Zhang Sanfeng*. (由 from 懂勁 Dong jin 而階及 step into 神明 Shén míng.)

《太極拳經 Tàijí quán jīng》張三丰 Zhang Sanfeng*

「...欲天下豪傑延年益壽，不徒作技藝之末也。」

" Tàijí quán jīng" Zhang Sanfeng* "... Tai chi is for the heroes of the world to achieve longevity, not only for martial arts , which is the least important aspect of tai chi. "https://zh.wikipedia.org/wiki/太極拳論

*張三丰 Zhang Sanfeng, his statue shown below was a legendary Chinese Taoist purported to have achieved immortality. He is said to be the legendary creator of tai chi when he saw a coiled up snake that could fought off its deadly predator, an eagle.

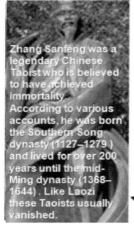

Zhang Sanfeng was a legendary Chinese Taoist who is believed to have achieved immortality. According to various accounts, he was born the Southern Song dynasty (1127–1279) and lived for over 200 years until the mid-Ming dynasty (1368–1644). Like Laozi these Taoists usually vanished.

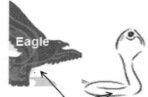

Eagle

A coiled up snake defeated its deadly predator, the eagle triggered the invention of tai chi by the Taoist, *Zhang Sanfeng*.

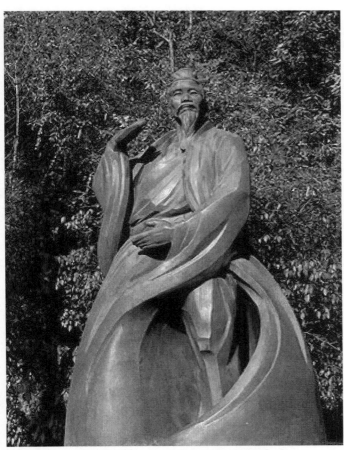

**By Gisling - Own work, CC BY 3.0,
https://commons.wikimedia.org/w/index.php?curid=85
30671**

9/Practicing the Nine Sessions Buddhist Wind Breathing,九節佛風 Jiǔ jié fú fēng is one of the ways to reach Shen ming:

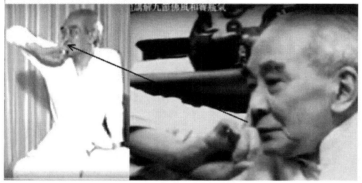

https://www.youtube.com/watch?v=Za0wxuF4ilg&index=9&lis
t=LLNg02k-r3xnmukgVFfPc-yA南老师示范九节佛风及宝瓶气
(Eng Sub) the 9 Sessions Buddhist Wind Breathing a super-
slow breathing.　　Master Nan demonstrates one form of
Integrative Mind Body Training (IMBT),.

The following instructions for the acquisition of Bǎo píng qì **寶瓶氣 are based on the following video:**

https://www.youtube.com/watch?v=pfe1-
qdrESQ&list=PLf1IA5I7JRuZmxNpbrmaRVnSO3i3-
6WKo

宝瓶气修法

In Tibetan Buddhism Bǎo píng qì **寶瓶氣 is an advanced form of breathing practice, similar to the Cháhú qì 茶壺氣 or píng qì 瓶氣 in yoga and Fēng lú 風爐 or liàndān lú 煉丹爐 in Daoism. When a practitioner succeeds in the acquisition of this state he or she requires very little breathing and**

his or her posture will be perfect and straight and he or she would not have to worry about a big stomach.

Instructions :

Assume the following sitting posture:

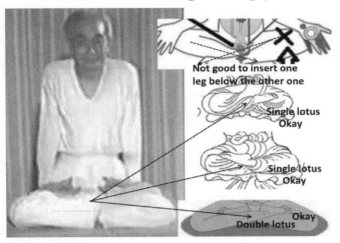

Not good to insert one leg below the other one

Single lotus
Okay

Single lotus
Okay

Okay
Double lotus

Configure the hands as shown in the picture and place them on the thighs as shown in the picture with the palms up. Straighten the elbows and raise both shoulders upwards.

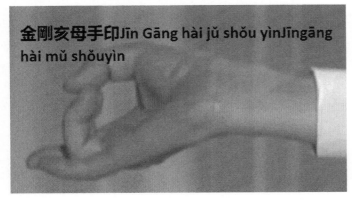

金剛亥母手印Jīn Gāng hài jǔ shǒu yìnJīngāng hài mǔ shǒuyìn

(Author's note: The purpose of this posture is to stretch up the spine and to stretch out the shoulder joints in order to strengthen the CranioSacral postural reflex of weightless feeling of the head and the abdominal part below the umbilicus sticking towards the spine.)

Use the nostrils to breathe in slowly until the maximum breathing capacity is reached. Hold the breath. The level of sophistication is counted by the number of beats. The duration of each beat is counted by the right hand hitting the right knee, then the left knee, then the forehead and a snap of the fingers. It is about 2 seconds. If you can hold the breath for the duration of 36 beats (36x2seconds=1 minute 12 seconds) you have reached the lowest rank of Bǎo píng qì 寶瓶氣. When you can last for 72 beats (2 minutes 24 seconds) you have advanced to the middle rank and when you can last for 108 (3 minutes 36 seconds) beats you have reached the top rank.

One important point:

The left nostril has to be functional when practicing Bǎo píng qì. If only the right nostril is functional do not practice Bǎo píng qì.

When you breathe in do it slowly with the lower abdomen. When you breathe out do it with some force and do it quickly. From my personal experiences if you have Qi Tie Bai 氣 貼 背 the adhesive feeling of the part below the umbilicus will become stronger during respiration. The lifting up of the shoulders with the straightened arms helps to stretch out the shoulder joints and to straighten the spine.

When this breathing practice is sophisticated the inhalation and exhalation gradually and naturally slow down and eventually become minimal. Your respiration becomes so slow observers might think you are not breathing. You will feel that your mind is clear without any disturbances from wondering thoughts. If you have the flu it can be cured by this physical mental condition. Your kung fu will becomes better and better when you can concentrate your mental calmness with the slow breathing.

《如何修證佛法》

Taoists have a similar breathing practice, called Embryonic respiration, Tai xi 胎息 in Chinese.

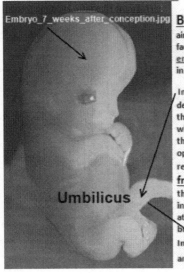

Embryo_7_weeks_after_conception.jpg

Umbilicus

Breathing is the process of moving air into and out of the lungs to facilitate gas exchange with the internal environment, mostly by bringing in oxygen and flushing out carbon dioxide.

In physiology, **respiration** is defined as the movement of oxygen from the outside environment to the cells within tissues, and the transport of carbon dioxide in the opposite direction. You could also define respiration as **the release of energy from glucose** and this is achieved through the breaking down of this glucose in the cells and oxygen from the atmosphere is absolutely pivotal to this breaking down.

In Chinese both Breathing and respiration are called 呼吸 Hūxī.

The illustrations in the picture have been enlarged in the following picture:

Breathing is the process of moving air into and out of the lungs to facilitate gas exchange with the internal environment, mostly by bringing in oxygen and flushing out carbon dioxide. le.

In physiology, **respiration** is defined as the movement of oxygen from the outside environment to the cells within tissues, and the transport of carbon dioxide in the opposite direction. You could also define respiration as **the release of energy from glucose** and this is achieved through the breaking down of this glucose in the cells and oxygen from the atmosphere is absolutely pivotal to this breaking down.

In Chinese both Breathing and respiration are called 呼吸 **Hūxī.**

According to the author of this paper's own experiences it is the best breathing practice when doing the sleeping qi gong of Master Chen Tuan.

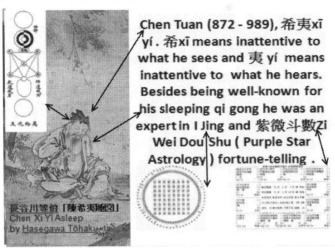

Chen Tuan (872 - 989), 希夷 xī yí . 希 xī means inattentive to what he sees and 夷 yí means inattentive to what he hears. Besides being well-known for his sleeping qi gong he was an expert in I Jing and 紫微斗數 Zi Wei Dou Shu (Purple Star Astrology) fortune-telling .

長谷川等伯「陳希夷圖引」
Chen Xi Yi Asleep
by Hasegawa Tōhaku

The illustrations in the picture have been enlarged in the following picture:

Chen Tuan (872 - 989), 希夷 xī yí . 希 xī means inattentive to what he sees and 夷 yí means inattentive to what he hears. Besides being well-known for his sleeping qi gong he was an expert in I Jing and 紫微斗數 Zi Wei Dou Shu (Purple Star Astrology) fortune-telling .

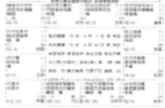

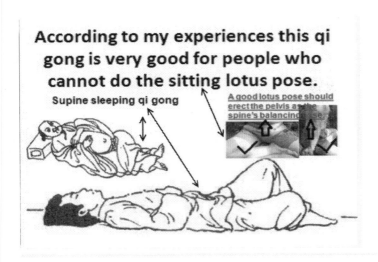

According to my experiences this qi gong is very good for people who cannot do the sitting lotus pose.

Supine sleeping qi gong

A good lotus pose should erect the pelvis as the spine's balancing base.

The illustrations in the picture have been enlarged in the following picture:

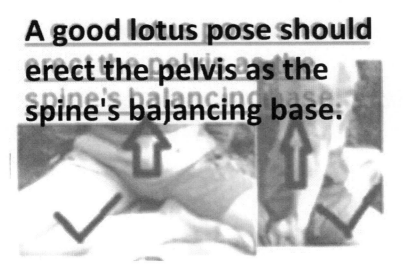

A good lotus pose should erect the pelvis as the spine's balancing base.

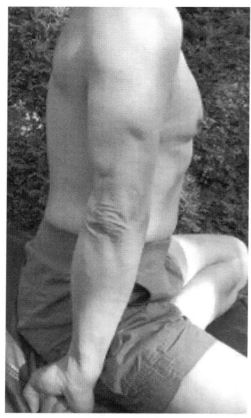

Please note the lumbar curve of the low back.

10/In another writing of Master Wǔ, "The explanation of the 13 Tai Chi moves 十三勢行功心解 Shísān shì xíng gōng xīn jiě", he said, "Each Tai Chi move is a cycle that should have a total body movement of muscle contraction and relaxation. His original wording is as followed, "往復須有摺疊=folding". The modern concept of alternative muscle contraction and relaxation to store and release power is better visualized by the analogy of a coiled spring instead of an arrow. The coiled spring analogy was used by Master Yǔxiāng Wǔ's contemporary, the Yang style Tai Chi family, in their secret instruction manual of the cultivation of the 8 basic forms of power in Tai Chi .

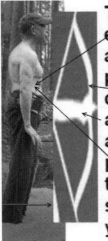

The ready posture to execute the Peng or any other form of tai chi power is like a slightly drawn bow with an arrow in a "song kai" and ready to store power state. Is it right to call this a "relaxed" state? Please make your own judgement.

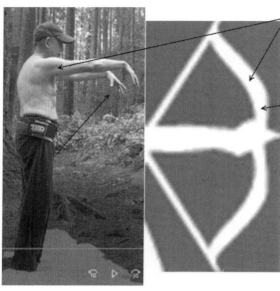

The Peng form of tai chi power is like a drawn bow with an adhesion to the oncoming force. It is ready to exert its power or to convert itself into a different form of tai chi power.

11/ The peng form of power is the first and the most important of the 8 basic forms of power in Tai Chi and these 8 basic forms of power have been vaguely explained in a set of definitions, kept as a top secret by the Yang style Tai Chi family for many years. The following is the exact quotation of the first of the 8 basic forms of power, "掤 (peng) 勁義何解? 如水負行舟,先實丹田氣,次要頂頭懸,全體彈簧力,開合一定間,任有千斤重飄浮亦不難". The following is my interpretation as an illustration of the meaning of jin in general and the peng form of power in particular. The peng form of power is like a boat floating on the water "如(like)水(water)負(carries)行舟(boat)". In the first move of any style of Tai Chi the arms that are raised to meet an imaginary oncoming force are the boats. Pictorial illustrations of the 8 basic forms of power in Tai Chi are illustrated further down in the article. To generate the peng form of power to do this movement one has to compress the Dantian first (the lower abdominal cavity) making it solid. "先 (firstly) 實 (making it solid) 丹田 (Dantian, the lower abdominal cavity) 氣 (qi)".Then (次) the head (頭) has to feel as light as if it was hanging (懸) in the air "次要頂頭懸". This means that the neck and the throat cavity have to be trained to become as solid as the abdominal cavity so that the body can move as a solid whole piece. This interpretation is a more concrete description of what Yǔxiāng Wǔ (武) said in his "The explanation of the 13 Tai Chi moves," that in a Tai Chi move one should move the body as a whole and stop the body's movements as a whole, "一動(move)無有不動，一靜(stillness)無有不靜".

Incidentally the throat, anatomically known as the pharyngeal space, is structurally similar to the abdominal Dantian. The skull is like an inverted sacrum and a consolidated pharyngeal cavity can support the head so well that it gives the individual the feeling that the head is as light as if it was hanging in the air. For a full explanation of this throat Dantian concept it needs a full article so that it can be thoroughly examined.

After one has acquired the dong jin coordination the whole body (全體) is connected like a coiled spring (彈簧) that can store power (力) and release power like a spring "全體彈簧力". Just like the action of a coiled spring, the power is released in a moment of stillness (一定間) during the opening (開) and closing (合) of the spring mechanism.

The stillness, Ding 定 in the moment of stillness (一定間) is a very important condition that must be practised and acquired in the preparatory pose of Tai Chi when the body is composed in a balanced manner and connected as a whole and in a ready position to move as a whole. The body in a condition of stillness could be used to store up power like a coiled spring when compressed. This power compression process is like submerging a ball into the water and the reactive buoyancy (浮) of the water gives the ball a strong power that can carry "a thousand catty of weight" (千斤重). "任有千斤重飄浮亦不難". The reactive buoyancy of the water is a good analogy of the Tai Chi practitioner's conscious efforts in the pile stance practice to employ as many muscles of the body as possible to react to the gravitational pull of the earth, which acts like the water that carries the boat "如水負行舟". In my article, mentioned at the beginning of this essay I have pointed out that the the peng form of power should not be translated as "warding off".

In Tai Chi, one uses the unique adhesive kung fu (沾連粘隨不丟頂) to make the opponent lose his or her balance and finish off the job with one or a mixture of the eight forms of power in Tai Chi. If an opponent is being "warded off" has he or she been off balance before or after the Tai Chi manoeuvre ? Where is the adhesive, the yin component, the power absorbing part of the Tai Chi circle? At the most "warding off" could only be regarded as the yang part of the Tai Chi cycle. The closest translation of 掤 I can think of is a fuzzily reactive and adhesive form of power.

12/ My complex translation of the peng form of power is consistent with the water buoyancy of a boat carrying weight. A boat in the water will not forcefully resist any weight added on it. It will give room for the weight and build up just enough resistance to deal with the problem. In Tai Chi when the weight is too much for the peng form of power alone to resist, other forms of power will be used to deal with the problem. This strategic manoeuvre of the 8 forms of Tai Chi power will be fully illustrated later in this article. However, it will be useless to practice the usage of these variations if one does not have the total body movements with the coordinating muscle connection of the whole body.

13/This kind of connecting the muscles of the total body movements, called the practice of pile standing can be practised by itself or at the beginning of a Tai Chi practice. It should be assumed at the beginning of any style of Tai Chi Chuan practice. Without any learned reflex most people just stand with the muscles of the legs and the feet. If you practised pile standing the way most people stand with only the muscles of the legs and feet you will never acquire this postural reflex that has to be learned. Pile stance should be trained the same way like training the peng form of power. To generate the peng form of power one has to compress the Dantian first (the abdominal cavity) making it solid.

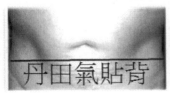

The black line shows a sign of my well-formed
← Dantian, with the abdominal part below the naval adhering towards the spine 丹田氣貼背)

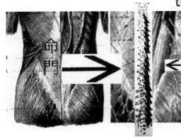

←The arrows show the Erector spinalis muscles (the Mingmen命門) that straightens up the back.

The above picture have been enlarged:

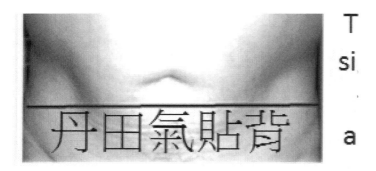

T

si

a

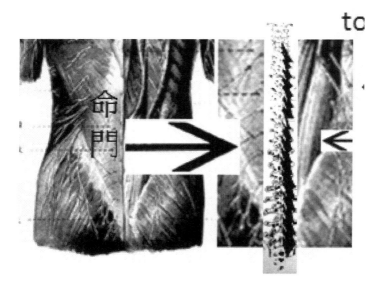

to

The black line shows a sign of my well-formed
← Dantian, with the abdominal part below the naval adhering towards the spine 丹田氣貼背)
←The arrows show the Erector spinalis muscles (the Mingmen命門) that straightens up the back.

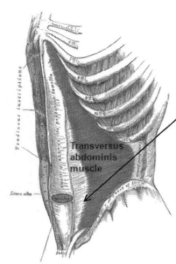

氣貼背 Qi tie (stick) bei (back) is the result of the lower part (below the umbilicus) of the Transversus abdominis muscle first contracts consciously and then it remains in the contracted state without any conscious effort. This feeling is hard to describe but once you get the reflex and you know what I mean. This is why I compare the tai chi CranioSacral postural reflex to learning how to ride a bicycle.

The illustrations in the abve picture have been enlarged in the following picture:

氣貼背 Qi tie (stick) bei (back) is the result of the lower part (below the umbilicus) of the Transversus abdominis muscle first contracts consciously and then it remains in the contracted state without any conscious effort. This feeling is hard to describe but once you get the reflex and you know what I mean. This is why I compare the tai chi CranioSacral postural reflex to learning how to ride a bicycle.

"先 (firstly) 實 (making it solid) 丹田 (Dantian, the abdominal cavity) 氣 (qi)".Then (次) the head (頭) has to feel as light as if it was hanging (懸) in the air "次要頂頭懸". This means that the neck and the throat cavity have to be as solid as the abdominal cavity so that the body becomes a solid whole piece and moves as a whole. Described in modern terminology pile stance training is a form of isometric muscle stimulation with the mental concentration to activate and recruit as many muscles as possible to respond to the newly learned postural reflex.

14/This is probably the best and the most integrative way to cure poor posture. This new interpretation opens up some new usages of Tai Chi. It can be used to treat poor posture, which is becoming epidemic with the new computer technology.

15/ The preparatory pose itself can be an effective form of exercise too. Macrae, F reported in *MailOnline* ;Dr Mike Loosemore, the Lead Consultant in Exercise Medicine at the Institute of Sport, Exercise and Health, says, 'The message I want to try to get out there is that small amounts of physical activity, although not reaching the government guidelines, are still doing you a lot of good – even just standing up is good for you. I'm standing up now, I'm using all the small muscles in my legs and the rest of me, I'm keeping myself upright. If I stood up like this and worked standing up, which I do, three hours a day, five days a week, that would be the equivalent of running ten marathons a year.' (Macrae, 2014) If ordinary standing can be an effective form of exercise can you imagine doing pile standing with many more postural muscles? People can use many short periods of free time to do this simple and effective exercise if they have acquired the Tai Chi CranioSacral postural reflex.

For a detailed explanation of my concept of the CranioSacral Postural reflex in Tai Chi please refer to my article, "<u>The CranioSacral postural reflex in Tai Chi Part 2:</u>" A brief introduction of this booklet series can be found in www.YouTube.com by searching with "CranioSacral postural reflex".

https://www.youtube.com/watch?v=LPbKYpoIMEU

The Tai Chi CranioSacral Postural Reflex for better posture and tai chi (Copyrights reserved)

My YouTube channel can be located by searching with "Dr. George Ho".

16/ In order to practice dong jin one of the prerequisites is to have acquired the physical condition as described by Master Chengfu Yang 楊澄甫 as "鬆開 Song kai". To practice "Song kai" you have to be in the Wuji 無極 state as described in 王宗岳 Zongyue Wang's 《太極拳論 *Tai Chi quán lùn*》, " 靜之則合*, the stable intertwined binary state of the yin and the yang." In concrete term it is the preparatory pose of any form of Tai Chi. When this simple pile standing pose is practised correctly over a period of time one could reach the following mind body condition as described by a well-known Tai Chi master, Master Peisheng Wang (1919- 2004), (王 p.19) "In order to excel in this preparatory pose one has to have a thoughtless and tranquil mind and a relaxed body. One has to have the feeling of standing on a mildly rocking boat; the body is swaying with the boat. Author's note: The body does not sway when practising this pose. With enough practice the mind-body complex has an indescribable comfortable feeling, which lasts till the end of practising the whole set of movements. This feeling can stay for a long time after practice. The longer it stays the better. It is for the mind and for health." The standing on rocking boat imagery is a vivid description of the use of the earth's gravitation pulling force to unify and align the muscles of the whole body into one direction. The reactive force of this downward pull is the upward buoyancy force that enables a boat to float on the water. This is one of the reasons why many Tai Chi teachers advise their students that after each session of practising their Tai Chi set they should stay motionless for a few minutes in the ending pose, which is the same as the preparatory pose. This pile standing practice will gradually enhance the reflexes acquired in the Tai Chi movement practice.

17/The slow Tai Chi set practice plays the role of enhancing and reinforcing the newly learned postural reflex so that it can be maintained during movements. The Tai Chi movements also serve the function of practicing the expression of the 8 forms of Tai Chi power and their combinations. In an ideal situation one can practice this kind of Integrative Body Mind Training (a scientific way to call Tai Chi) at any time when circumstances permit. Once the dong jin state has been reached every movement or stillness can be readily recalled in the dong jin state and this is why the ancient text claims that the don jin state is crucial for a continuous qualitative improvement of one's Tai Chi kung fu, which is not just the practice of the slow moving set. From personal experiences I can do this Integrative Body Mind Training in any body position, lying down or sitting. After I have acquired the state of dong jin it becomes a lot easier to enter the state of stillness, described in the Yang style Tai Chi's secret practice manual as the moment of stillness 一定間. If you just move slowly in your Tai Chi practice and do not move the body as a whole as specified in the definitions of the Yang style Tai Chi family's 8 basic forms of power you will never acquire the reflexes of a Tai Chi master. I shall use the analogy of riding a tricycles and a bicycle to illustrate my point. In appearance both forms of riding a vehicle of transportation are very similar. They both perform the same function. However the practice of riding on a tricycle will never get you any closer to acquiring the reflex of riding a bicycle. I hope this will clarify my claim that Tai Chi is not just moving slowly. Also after you have acquired the CranioSacral Postural reflex in Tai Chi you are another step closer to dong jin. In the following series of pictures I shall demonstrate all the 8 basic forms of power in Tai Chi. When you have a good understanding of these 8 basic forms of power of Tai Chi you will have a much better chance of acquiring the state of dǒng jìn.....

18/The peng form of power, demonstrated by Dr. George Ho in June, 2014:

The preparatory pose of any style of tai chi is demonstrated in the picture below.

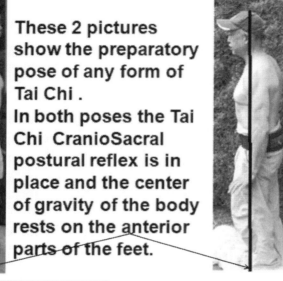

These 2 pictures show the preparatory pose of any form of Tai Chi .
In both poses the Tai Chi CranioSacral postural reflex is in place and the center of gravity of the body rests on the anterior parts of the feet.

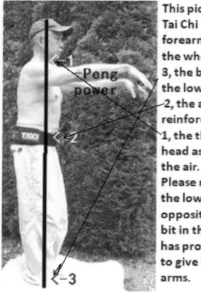

This picture shows the peng form of Tai Chi power expressed in the two forearms with power gathered from the whole body, starting from 3, the bottom of the feet, through the lower limbs into 2, the abdominal Dantian and reinforced by 1, the throat Dantian that makes the head as light as if it was hanging in the air.
Please note that the Mingmen of the lower back around the area opposite the umbilicus is caved in a bit in the preparatory pose and it has protruded slightly out in order to give better support to the two arms.

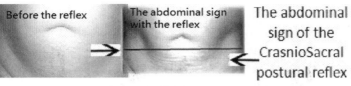

Before the reflex | The abdominal sign with the reflex

The abdominal sign of the CrasnioSacral postural reflex

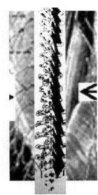

The 大明咒 mantra (Oṃ) (ma) (ṇi) (pad) (me) (hūṃ)

singing pauses at this (hūṃ) end for breathing in and the Mingmen muscles occasionally relax at this point.

In these two poses the most important training is in activating as many muscles as possible to do the job. The logic is very simple. When there are more people doing the job, it becomes easier.

Many Tai Chi teachers prescribe pile stance training quantitatively, like how many minutes in the beginning and which part of the body has to be in line with which part of the body. This is the traditional Chinese way of teaching. This tradition was functional in ancient China when social and group interests overruled individual rights. There is a very good reason for the formation of this tradition in ancient China when resources were scarce. After you have learned the rationale of why it had to be done this way you will agree with me that the traditional way may not be the best for our modern age of abundance that allows the flourishing of individual creativity that opens up new and innovative ways to make life better and more beautiful.

In ancient China many villages taught martial arts to all the men in the village. It was very hard for the teacher to give individual attention to this large group of students. With the rigid and easily observable objective and quantitative guidelines the gifted ones could be easily and objectively spotted. Those who could conform to the postural requirements and could stand for a long time without trouble were the best of that group. These selected ones had to go through specific rituals to make sure of their loyalty to the teacher (sifu). Then they were taught the real kung fu. Most sifus taught their real kung fu only to their sons. Many Tai Chi fans must have heard of the story that the founder of Yang style Tai Chi pretended that he was mute in order to gain the trust of the Chen Tai Chi family to let him worked as a servant and that was how he secretly observed and learned his Tai Chi kung fu without any direct teaching from any of the Chen family members. I am sure most people will agree with me that the Yang style Tai Chi kung fu is as good as the Chen style Tai Chi. In many forms of art there is only so much the teacher can teach. If the student does not have the artistic talent he or she cannot be an artist. One example is the Yang style Tai Chi. They kept their training very secretive. However, after three generations of keeping the leader status within the Yang family the representative status of the Yang style of Tai Chi went to a sifu unrelated to the Yang family.

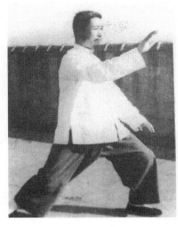

鄭曼青師承楊澄
甫,鄭老師是楊家太
極第四代代表

Master Man-ching <u>Cheng</u> is the 4th generation representative of the Yang style Tai chi

Master Man-ching Cheng 曼青鄭 taught in Taiwan and New York and was more famous than Master Chengfu Yang's son, Shǒu-zhōng Yang (1910-1985) who was teaching in Hong Kong. One of my friends who went to Shǒu-zhōng Yang's lessons was not impressed because he told me his push hand techniques were not as good as his wife. It was not an accident that other martial artists in Hong Kong picked and challenged Shǒu-zhōng Yang's Tai Chi competitor, Gōngyí Wú, the gate keeper of Wu style Tai Chi in a real public arena fight in Macau.

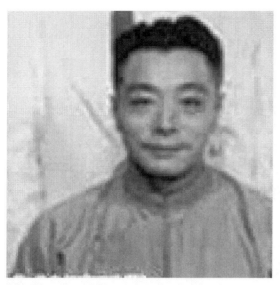

Gōngyí Wú 吳公儀

Everybody including the Wu style family members admitted that the founder of Wu's Tai Chi learned from the founder of Yang's Tai Chi. It is the singer not the song that makes the real difference in any kind of performance art. I hope this background information can convince many people that when learning Chinese art the traditional way may not be the easiest way to excel in that form of art. The Yang Tai Chi family's loss of its leader status shows us the so-called family secret is not a sure way to excel in these traditional ancient Chinese forms of art.

19/Because of China's deep cultural influence most Chinese have been somewhat conditioned to think that the traditional or the secret teachings are the guarantee of their success in learning that form of art.

As a Western trained health care professional I believe in the scientific ways and would try my best to gear my instructions according to individual differences.

For instance the objective way to monitor your pile stance is to compare the length of time you can stand without fatigue. One should not be told to persist for a definite time period. The scientific training way would make sure that everyone will succeed in getting the reflex. First, find out the maximum of time one can practice the pile stance and no one should practice beyond the point of fatigue. Then train to stand within 60-80% of the time frame of one's maximum capacity. Make sure protein in the form of meat or protein powder is ingested 30 minutes before or after the standing practice because the muscles need amino acids to build new muscle fibers. Then the progress in the practice of pile stance can be compared and monitored by the maximum capacity of the time one can practice without fatigue. The longer you can stand without getting tired the more muscles you have recruited and the stronger they have become.

In order to monitor your peng form of power objectively you can ask someone to hold your hands while you are in the preparatory pose and you try to raise your arms. If you only use the shoulder muscles, you probably cannot raise the person who holds your hands down with the weight of his or her body. If you have the CranioSacral postural Tai Chi reflex and have recruited the whole-body muscles to do this job you can easily raise your arms against the resistance. Most accomplished Tai Chi masters can perform this task without any problem. There is no magic and no trick and I have just told you my scientific explanation. When you have recruited more muscles to do the job it becomes easier.

In the picture below

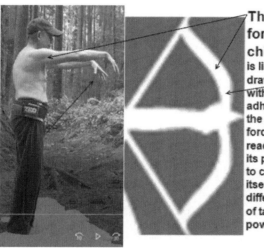

The Peng form of tai chi power is like a drawn bow with an adhesion to the oncoming force. It is ready to exert its power or to convert itself into a different form of tai chi power.

if you just use the shoulder muscles to raise the arms you are not practicing tai chi because in any tai chi move the movement is executed by the total body movements that resemble a snake.

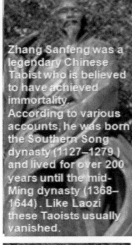

Zhang Sanfeng was a legendary Chinese Taoist who is believed to have achieved immortality. According to various accounts, he was born the Southern Song dynasty (1127–1279) and lived for over 200 years until the mid-Ming dynasty (1368–1644). Like Laozi these Taoists usually vanished.

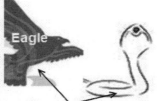

Eagle

A coiled up snake defeated its deadly predator, the eagle triggered the invention of tai chi by the Taoist, *Zhang Sanfeng.*

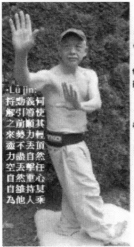

Lǚ jin:
持勁義词
解引等使
之前順其
來勢力輕
壺不丟頂
力盡自然
空丟擊往
自然重心
自雛持勁
為他人來

This is the lǚ form of tai chi power that changes from the peng form of power. The opponent is being "lǚed" up and out. Lǚ jin 持勁 is to use the adhesive force to direct the opponent's oncoming force to continue in the same direction to the extent that the opponent loses his or her balance. When the opponent has lost his or her balance and control you can launch your advance or aggression in whatever way you want. However you have to keep your balance to guard against the proponent's sudden attack from an adverse condition. For someone who knows the 8 forms of tai chi power there are at least 4 basic forms of power that can attack from an adverse condition. They will be illustrated later in this article.

The illustrations in the picture have been enlarged in the following picture:

This is the lǔ form of tai chi power that changes from the peng form of power. The opponent is being "lǔed" up and out. Lǔ jìn 捋勁 is to use the adhesive force to direct the opponent's oncoming force to continue in the same direction to the extent that the opponent loses his or her balance. When the opponent has lost his or her balance and control you can launch your advance or aggression in whatever way you want. However you have to keep your balance to guard against the proponent's sudden attack from an adverse condition. For someone who knows the 8 forms of tai chi power there are at least 4 basic forms of power that can attack from an adverse condition. They will be illustrated later in this article.

The 擠 Ji power is often used by many famous masters in demonstrations to throw people up in the air as seen in the Youtube video, 鄭曼青- 推手 (A Yang style master, *Zhèng Mànqīng – push hand*; the link is in the illustrations down below.) at 2.37.

I have seen a lot of injuries from tai chi push hand. In my article I have better ways to train and to evaluate one's tai chi power than to push people.

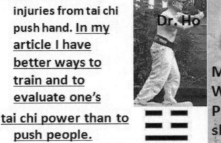
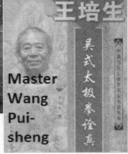

The trigram, 震 Zhèn☳

Jǐ jìn:擠勁義何解用時有兩方直接單純意迎合一動中間接反應力如球撞壁還又如錢投鼓躍然擊鏗鏘

Jǐ jìn has two methods in application. The first method is to meet the oncoming force and deflect it into a different direction so that it will not hit you. Another method is to deflect it right back to the opponent like a ball hitting the wall and being bounced back, or throwing a coin to a drum and the coin is bounced back with a loud sound. A better example for the first method is hitting the tennis ball on the rise in tennis.

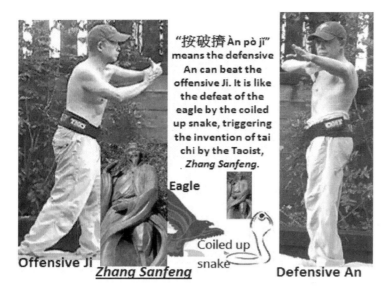

"按破擠 Àn pò jì" means the defensive An can beat the offensive Ji. It is like the defeat of the eagle by the coiled up snake, triggering the invention of tai chi by the Taoist, *Zhang Sanfeng*.

Eagle

Coiled up snake

Offensive Ji

Zhang Sanfeng

Defensive An

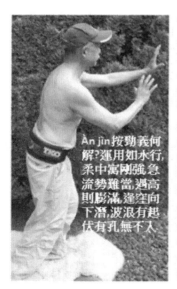

An jin 按勁義何解?運用如水行,柔中寓剛強,急流勢難當,遇高則膨滿,逢空向下潛,波浪有起伏,有孔無不入

The English translation of the Chinese instruction of an jin is as followed, "Àn jìn is like the running water of a rapid river in which the soft water becomes very strong. It rises up against any barrier and fills any empty space. Its hitting direction can be straight like the running river water. It can also be in a wavy form, using the change of direction to enhance its power at the angle of directional change. Àn jìn will fill any area of weakness of the opponent like water will fill any hole."

The illustrations in the picture have been enlarged in the following picture:

The English translation of the Chinese instruction of an jin is as followed, "Àn jìn is like the running water of a rapid river in which the soft water becomes very strong. It rises up against any barrier and fills any empty space. Its hitting direction can be straight like the running river water. It can also be in a wavy form, using the change of direction to enhance its power at the angle of directional change. Àn jìn will fill any area of weakness of the opponent like water will fill any hole."

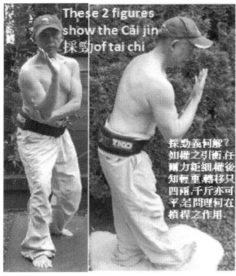

These 2 figures show the Căi jìn 採勁 of tai chi

採勁義何解？
如槓之引衡,任
兩力鉅細權後
知輕重,轉移只
四兩,千斤亦可
平若問理何在
槓桿之作用.

The English translation of Căi jìn 採勁 in Chinese is, "Căi jìn is the use of leverage so that a smaller force can manipulate a bigger force. The most important part is the ability to read the oncoming force's direction and forcefulness."

It is often used together with jǐ jìn, which deflects an oncoming force at the angle of directional change of the àn jìn

From personal experiences căi jìn is often used in a sudden attack in the form of jerking the arm or the hand of the opponent. As a chiropractor I have seen quite a few cases of whiplash injuries of the neck when the patient's arm is being jerked downward by his or her push hand partner, causing a car-crash kind of whiplash injury of the neck. This happens often in push-hand practices.

However, I have also adopted this form of Tai Chi power in my chiropractic manipulation. I have found it very effective to adjust the elbow joint for the treatment of tennis elbow. It is also very effective when used to reduce cervical (neck) disc herniation, which is often caused by a whiplash-kind of injury. Most chiropractic adjustment techniques are delivered in an explosive force of low amplitude and high velocity. Căi jìn is perfect for doing most chiropractic joint manipulation techniques. I think Tai Chi teachers who teach pushing hand techniques should try to acquire a license to do therapy so that they can treat injuries during practice immediately. Fresh injuries are a lot easier to treat because inflammation has not occurred yet. Without the damages caused by inflammation they heal a lot faster. A good marketing technique for any Tai Chi school is to have an in-house chiropractic clinic with a chiropractor available for on the spot and immediate treatments for push hand injuries.

Zhou is an offensive move. When the fist strike misses and you have lost your balance because of the miss, attack with the elbow to regain your balance and to enhance the power with the sudden stop of the fall momentum. Please examine the gen trigram with a solid yang stroke of the upper body and the lower 2 strokes are the broken yin strokes. The power generated by the front leg's solid step on the ground to regain balance reinforces the union of the hand and the shoulder acupuncture points. This is the message conveyed by the gen trigram.

Zhou肘, cai採, kao靠 and lie挒 are the 4 brisk forms of power of tai chi. I have found this high velocity brisk form of power very useful in my chiropractic manipulation.

The trigram gen ☶ is like an overturned bowl.

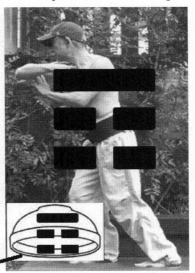

The illustrations in the picture have been enlarged in the following picture:

Zhou is an offensive move. When the fist strike misses and you have lost your balance because of the miss, attack with the elbow to regain your balance and to enhance the power with the sudden stop of the fall momentum. Please examine the gen trigram with a solid yang stroke of the upper body and the lower 2 strokes are the broken yin strokes. The power generated by the front leg's solid step on the ground to regain balance reinforces the union of the hand and the shoulder acupuncture points. This is the message conveyed by the gen trigram.

Zhou肘, cai採, kao靠 and lie挒 are the 4 brisk forms of power of tai chi. I have found this high velocity brisk form of power very useful in my chiropractic manipulation.

The trigram gen ☶ is like an overturned bowl.

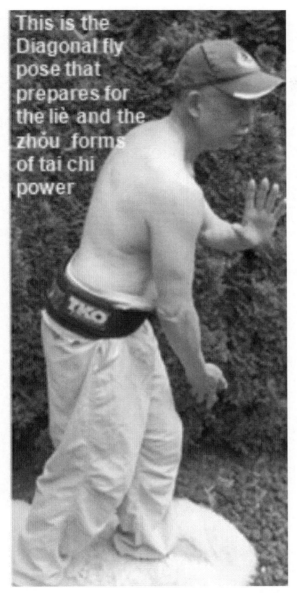

This is the Diagonal fly pose that prepares for the liè and the zhŏu forms of tai chi power

I also encourage the acquisition of Tai Chi's 8 basic forms of power for chiropractors and other health care professionals who do joint manipulation or medical procedures that require this kind of explosive burst of power. They will find that practicing Tai Chi is good for their health and their practice. For instance, they can do group therapy to treat poor posture with the instructions to acquire the Tai Chi CranioSacral Postural reflex. This will open up a new way to use Tai Chi for health. I have found the use of căi jìn in manipulation very useful in my 30 years of chiropractic practice. If there is any alternative medicine school that is interested in this suggestion I can put together a special training program for their students. For the time being I call this "Health Enhancement with the Tai Chi CranioSacral Postural Reflex".

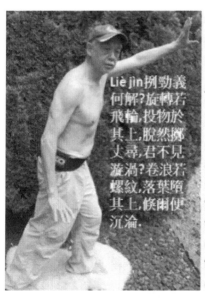

The English translation of Liè jìn is as followed, "Liè jìn can be visualized if you imagine the centrifugal force of a flywheel or a swirl. The spinning force generated by this move is the centrifugal force that hits the opponent."

This is the end move of the Diagonal fly pose at the completion of the liè form of tai chi power.

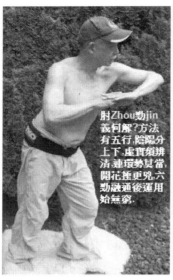

肘Zhòu勁jìn義何解?方法有五行,陰陽分上下,虛實須拼清,連環勢其當,開花捶更兇,六勁融通後運用始無窮.

Zhǒu jìn is literally the use of the elbow to hit the weakness of the opponent who is too close to be hit with the fist. Once you have created enough distance the fist can follow as the second blow. However you have to have a good understanding of all the aforementioned forms of power and have to be able ti incorporate them with this zhǒu jìn then the applications have unlimited potentials of variations.

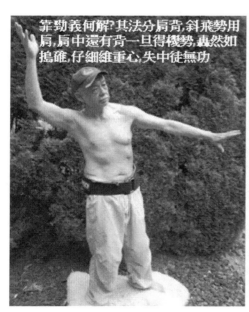

靠勁義何解?其法分肩背,斜飛勢用肩,肩中還有背一旦得機勢,轟然如搗碓,仔細維重心,失中徒無功

Kào jìn 靠勁 is best visualized in the diagonal flying move in Tai Chi. The shoulder is used to hit the opponent like a pestle pounding rice or garlic in the mortar. The back can be used after the shoulder misses the opponent. But you have to maintain your balance.

Of all the 8 basic forms of power the peng form of power is the most important and it is unique

when compared to other forms of martial arts s. If you have a good understanding and control of using the peng form of power and know how to integrate it with the other seven forms of Tai Chi power using the muscles of the whole body you have reached the state of dong jin. However, the Tai Chi movement practice has to be complemented with a slow pattern of breathing so that the body and mind can be trained as a whole. Breathing is the important link between the mind and the body. This has been scientifically explained in a modern investigation, called the Integrative Mind Body Training. The aforementioned 9 sessions Buddhist wind breathing 九節佛風 Jiǔ jié fú fēng is a good example of breathing training in an IMBT fashion.

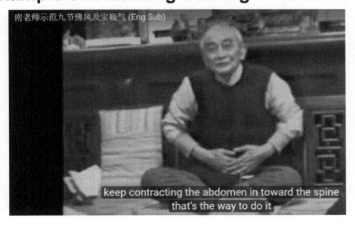

南老师示范九节佛风及宝瓶气 (Eng Sub)

keep contracting the abdomen in toward the spine
that's the way to do it

Singing is the art of breathing in:

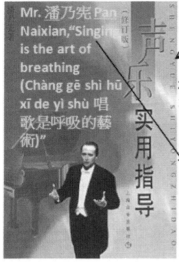

Mr. 潘乃宪 Pan Naixian, "Singing is the art of breathing (Chàng gē shì hū xī de yì shù 唱歌是呼吸的藝術)"

Practical Instructions for Vocalists (shēngyuè shíyòng zhǐdǎo) **published by** 上海音乐出版社, **in 1994 written by a famous Chinese music teacher,**

Mr. 潘乃宪 Pan Naixian

20/I have found that Dantian singing in Chinese opera is another way. It is more objectively observable because the progress in singing and chanting can be easily observed, recorded and compared. It can be practiced anytime anywhere on your own without a partner. It can be combined with any movement practice. The acting and singing in Chinese opera is a good example. 李海泉 Lee Moon-shuen (1901 – 1965) known professionally as Lee Hoi-chuen, was a Hong Kong Cantonese opera singer and film actor. He was the father of Bruce Lee.

https://en.wikipedia.org/wiki/Lee_Hoi-chuen

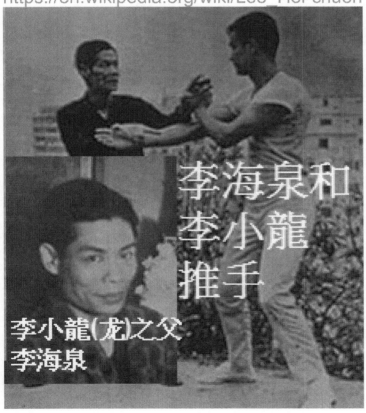

21/I have combined Dantian singing with my Dolphin Instant tai chi (The introductory YouTube movie is called, "Dolphin Instant Tai Chi".) when I swim and Treadmill Ram Tai Chi (The introductory YouTube movie is called, "Walk and chant into Chan ding (Samadhi) for health and longevity by Huai-jin Nan and Dr. George Ho".) with my hiking.

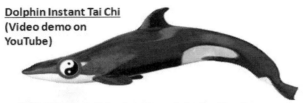

Dolphin Instant Tai Chi
(Video demo on
YouTube)

- A **scientifically explained** way to apply the health enhancement mechanisms of this empirically based ancient Chinese martial art.
- Effective for:
- **Posture correction and better voice** support by a consolidated belly way of breathing. When combined with a customised diet this will **reduce belly fat** and is conducive in the treatment and prevention of cardiovascular and diabetic problems. This exercise plan can **complement any form of therapy**.
- Written by **Dr. George Ho**

The illustrations in the picture have been enlarged in the following picture:

A **scientifically explained** way to apply the health enhancement mechanisms of this empirically based ancient Chinese martial art.

Effective for:

Posture correction and better voice support by a consolidated belly way of breathing. When combined with a customised diet this will **reduce belly fat** and is conducive in the treatment and prevention of cardiovascular and diabetic problems. This exercise plan can **complement any form of therapy**.

Written by **Dr. George Ho**

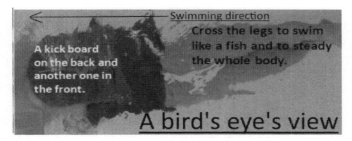

Swimming direction
Cross the legs to swim like a fish and to steady the whole body.

A kick board on the back and another one in the front.

A bird's eye's view

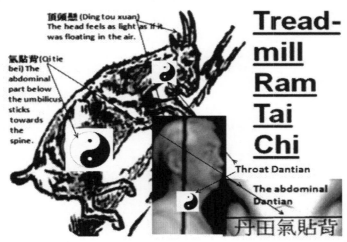

頂頸懸 (Ding tou xuan) The head feels as light as if it was floating in the air.

氣貼背(Qi tie bei) The abdominal part below the umbilicus sticks towards the spine.

Tread-mill Ram Tai Chi

Throat Dantian

The abdominal Dantian

丹田氣貼背

"Walk and chant into Chan ding (Samadhi) for health and longevity by Huai-jin Nan and Dr. George Ho"

....

Bibliography:

培生, 王. *吳式太极拳诠真*. 1st. Beijing: 人民体育出版社, 2003. .print.

懷瑾, 南.*如何修證佛法*.臺北.老古文化事業股份有限公司. (1996). print

(Macrae, 2014) *MailOnline - news, sport, celebrity, science and health stories Read more: http://www.dailymail.co.uk/health/article-2663889/Standing-three-hours-day-health-benefits-10-marathons-says-leading-doctor.html*

My books in Amazon.ca can be searched at:
https://www.amazon.ca/s/ref=nb_sb_noss_1?url=search-alias%3Daps&field-keywords=george+ho
1.The Dantian's Anatomy and Functions Explained Medically by Dr. George Ho
The link to the ebook in Amazon.ca followed by the abstract of this ebook:
https://www.amazon.ca/dp/B07GSJT8G7/ref=sr_1_2?ie=UTF8&qid=1535075597&sr=8-2&keywords=george+ho
Related supplemental YouTube video:
https://www.youtube.com/watch?v=LXuOjJfQ_Vc&index=8&list=PL9RRMUY60ixRHjIpvRSXudWjBVJF2rbkF

2.Can Tai Chi be self-learned? (Tai Chi and meditation by Dr. George Ho Book 1)
The link to this book:
https://www.amazon.ca/Benefits-tai-chi-spine-CranioSacral-ebook/dp/B07D8GVFCY/ref=sr_1_6?ie=UTF8&qid=1530421365&sr=8-6&keywords=george+ho
Related supplemental YouTube video:
https://www.youtube.com/watch?v=xQK0EnXWz4M&list=PL9RRMUY60ixRHjIpvRSXudWjBVJF2rbkF&index=2

Self-taught tai chi? Answer in Kindle by Dr. George Ho

3.The Benefits of tai chi for the spine: The postural enhancement effect of tai chi, called the CranioSacral Postural reflex of Tai Chi (Tai chi and meditation Book 2)
The link to this book:
https://www.amazon.ca/Benefits-tai-chi-spine-CranioSacral-ebook/dp/B07D8GVFCY/ref=sr_1_3?s=digital-text&ie=UTF8&qid=1537985769&sr=1-3&keywords=george+ho
Related supplemental YouTube video:
4.The path to Enlightenment from the practice of Tai Chi + 站椿 Zhàn zhuāng (pile stance): Shen Ming is the Enlightenment Stage of Tai Chi, Superior to the ... Dong Jin" (tai chi and meditation Book 3)
The link to this book:
The path to Enlightenment from the practice of Tai Chi + 站椿 Zhàn zhuāng (pile stance): The Shen Ming of Tai Ch is the complementary component of your meditation for Enlightenment
https://www.amazon.ca/Enlightenment-practice-站椿 Zhàn-zhuāng-stance/dp/1983262641/ref=sr_1_10?ie=UTF8&qid=1537985438&sr=8-10&keywords=george+ho
Related supplemental YouTube video:
https://www.youtube.com/watch?v=CRpFxoWD41w&index=4&list=PL9RRMUY60ixRHjIpvRSXudWjBVJF2rbkF

The path to Enlightenment from the practice of Tai Chi + 站椿 Zhàn zhuāng (pile stance)

5.Treadmill Ram Tai Chi (TRTC): Chan (Zen in Japanese) walking with the breathing practice for health and longevity by Huai-jin Nan and Dr. George Ho (tai chi and meditation Book 4) The link to this book: https://www.amazon.ca/Treadmill-Ram-Tai-Chi-TRTC-ebook/dp/B07GJXGMWZ/ref=sr_1_5?s=digital-text&ie=UTF8&qid=1537985769&sr=1-5&keywords=george+ho The related supplemental YouTube video: https://www.youtube.com/watch?v=qEGjemhyvNc&index=1&list=PL9RRMUY60ixRHjIpvRSXudWjBVJF2rbkF

Chan (Zen in Japanese) walking can enhance the function of the kidneys

https://www.youtube.com/watch?v=UwJW0rjUkFY&list=PL9RRMUY60ixRHjIpvRSXudWjBVJF2rbkF&index=3

6.The Ji 挤 form of tai chi power compared with Bruce Lee's One-in-punch: The Ji 挤 form of tai chi power explained and trained scientifically (tai chi and meditation Book 5) The link to this book: https://www.amazon.ca/Benefits-tai-chi-spine-CranioSacral-ebook/dp/B07D8GVFCY/ref=sr_1_3?s=digital-text&ie=UTF8&qid=1537985769&sr=1-3&keywords=george+ho **Related supplemental YouTube video:** https://www.youtube.com/watch?v=51-pTS2-JxM&list=PL9RRMUY60ixRHjIpvRSXudWjBVJF2rbkF&index=6

The Ji 挤 form of tai chi power compared with Bruce Lee's One-in-punch

7.Dolphin Instant Tai Chi This link to this book:

https://www.amazon.ca/Dolphin-Instant-Tai-Chi-George-ebook/dp/B07G459TYR/ref=sr_1_8?s=digital-text&ie=UTF8&qid=1537985769&sr=1-8&keywords=george+ho
Related supplemental YouTube video:
https://www.youtube.com/watch?v=mK8pnjf_hDQ&index=5&list=PL9RRMUY60ixRHjIpvRSXudWjBVJF2rbkF

THE EASIEST TAI CHI TO LEARN, "Dolphin Instant Tai Chi"

8.Meditation Bliss and Physical Health with Chan Walking and Swimming for All, including the Disabled

Amazon.ca's Kindle book link:

https://www.amazon.ca/dp/B07H1NWB51/ref=sr_1_2?ie=UTF

8&qid=1535947626&sr=8-2&keywords=george+ho☐

Related supplemental YouTube video:
https://www.youtube.com/watch?v=4HlvOa2XLkc&list=PL9RRMUY60ixRHjIpvRSXudWjBVJF2rbkF&index=9

Meditation Bliss and Physical Health with Chan Walking and Swimming for All, including the Disabled

9.Prof. Lin Jùnqīng's 8 Steps of the Pharyngeal Voice Training 林俊卿博士（咽音練聲法的八個步驟）

The link to this book: https://www.amazon.ca/Prof-Jùnqīngs-Steps-Pharyngeal-Training-ebook/dp/B07HDYSW5H/ref=sr_1_1?s=digital-text&ie=UTF8&qid=1537985769&sr=1-1&keywords=george+ho

His writing in Chinese is available free on the internet by searching with " 林俊卿博士（咽音練聲法的八個步驟）"□
Related supplemental YouTube video:
Kindle: Prof. Lin Jùnqīng's 8 Steps of the Pharyngeal Voice Training 林俊卿博士（咽音練聲法的八個步驟）

Prof. Line's original writing has been translated into English by Dr. George Ho of Vancouver and it has been published in Kindle.

10.The rehab exercise for "TFCC self-treatment" ebook at Amazon.ca by Dr. George Ho

The link to this book: https://www.amazon.ca/TFCC-Self-treatment-George-Kam-Ho-ebook/dp/B07D278WVV/ref=sr_1_11?s=digital-text&ie=UTF8&qid=1537985769&sr=1-11&keywords=george+ho

Related supplemental YouTube video:
https://www.youtube.com/watch?v=b_Ox_HaZSc0
The rehab exercise for "TFCC self-treatment" ebook at Amazon.ca by Dr. George Ho

11. The Correct Interpretations of Two Important Tai Chi Concepts: "鬆開 Song kai" by Yang Chengfu 楊澄甫 and Peng jin 弸 勁, the Peng form of concentrated Tai Chi power
12. The Guidelines for Self-taught Tai Chi and Sleeping Qigong (Kindle book)
https://www.youtube.com/watch?v=GQe01SUB2n8
The link to the book at Amazon.ca:
https://www.amazon.ca/dp/B07K5FXZ8B/ref=sr_1_2?ie=UTF8 &qid=1541281936&sr=8-2&keywords=george+ho☐

Dr. George Ho's publications in English:
I have the following articles in scanned pdf format available online.
Articles in English:

To buy the article pay US$ 5 to the PayPal account, Georgekwho@gmail.com. After payment the article in scanned pdf format will be sent out by e-mail from Vancouver:
1/ "A Non-invasive Cure of Plantar Fasciitis" (All copyrights reserved)
https://www.youtube.com/watch?v=2J_HQ9y2xOM
2/"A Non-drug, Non-surgery Tennis Elbow Cure"
https://www.youtube.com/watch?v=9g7gjWw0JyY&index=5&list=PL9RRMUY60ixTvXmr6dKYQU9GGdhx-7G1n
3/ "The Innovative Self-management of Sacroiliac joint dysfunction; one-sided buttock back pain"
https://www.youtube.com/watch?v=NGL4G0kMSVg&index=6&list=PL9RRMUY60ixTvXmr6dKYQU9GGdhx-7G1n

My Youtube channel:
Thanks you all for this 2943 subscriber's mile stone of my YouTube channel with   430,761 views and 2627 likes reached on 18th Nov., 2016.
The top ten movies getting some of the 2627 likes are:
1/Non-invasive cure of the piriformis syndrome by PNF (Copyrights reserved)
135 likes
2/(2)The Sacroiliac Joint Dysfunction Cure with an Innovative and Safe Self Treatment
55like
3/The tai chi 1/ 掤勁(1/Peng jin)Peng power (energy) explained in the mystical dimension of Yi Jing 易經
67likes

4/Curing lumbar disc hernia and acute low back pain (All copyrights reserved)
35 likes
5/The Dantian training secret in the old Cantonese opera tradition by Dr. George Ho
30 likes
6/(1 knee care) Smart care of the knee in exercises like Tai Chi and Qi gong
27 likes
7/The tai chi 2/ 捋勁 (2/Lu jin) Lu power (energy) explained in the mystical dimension of Yi Jing 易經
21likes
8/Practicing the first 5 basic forms of tai chi power with the 6 Healing sounds
19 likes
9/A supplemental movie to my first article of my Dantian and Mingmen' series (All copyrights reserved)
19 likes
10/Rejuvenation (4) Interpreting Master Huai-jin Nan's Anapana breathing technique
19 likes
A sequel to "Non-invasive cure of the piriformis syndrome by PNF stretching"(Copyrights reserved)
18 likes
The most popular playlists are:
  1/Tai Chi, Dantian and Mingmen
2/Dr. George Ho - English videos
3/The 8 forms of power (also been translated as energy) of tai chi
感謝大家的捧場,在下的 YouTube 頻道超越了 2900 定閱者的里程碑,

• 想自療以下健康問題者,請購買在下的文章, 線上購買文章(scanned pdf format) 途徑: 費用:美金 US$5 元,用 PayPal a/c:, 付款給 Georgekwho@gmail.com,收到付款+電郵地址後便從溫哥華電郵出文章。可通過電郵 Georgekwho@gmail.com 接觸筆者。

•

第一篇文章

治大肚腩: 1/"丹田、命門的生理解剖和練法介紹: 以氣的科學定義解釋為何太極名師多大肚腩(練丹田的壞副作用)?及防治大肚腩方法

"https://www.youtube.com/watch?v=TusZYhsxABA&list=TLGQaXtuokbNs

第 2 篇文章

治足底筋膜炎: 購買每一篇文章(scanned pdf format) 途徑: 購買自療足底筋膜炎

https://www.youtube.com/watch?v=LJ8h1RP7Le8&list=TLGQaXtuokbNs

第 3 篇教減肥

治高血壓高血糖: /"非藥物高血壓高血糖綜合療法"已出版兩篇文章

• **https://www.youtube.com/watch?v=um0F3H8sTFA**

第 4 篇文章

治媽媽手,腱鞘炎: 文章名:治媽媽手,腱鞘炎,購文章途徑

https://www.youtube.com/watch?v=84VVEoZuVrg&list=TLGQaXtuokbNs

第 5 篇文章

治尾指側手腕痛: "非手術非藥物尾指 側手腕痛自療法

https://www.youtube.com/watch?v=smbv9wxxfc8

第 6 篇文章解釋

練太極拳治壞姿勢之原理: "氣貼背頂頭懸合乎現代醫學解釋之丹田強脊健體法"

https://www.youtube.com/watch?v=9GPPO2UugGI

第 7 篇文章治單側腰眼部位的腰痛: :"創新非手術非藥物骶髂關節綜合症結合診斷治療的療法

"https://www.youtube.com/watch?v=aIjQXJ3NZxo

https://www.youtube.com/watch?v=rD_5ADuR48Y

第 8 篇文章

治網球肘: 網球肘綜合療法

"https://www.youtube.com/watch?v=Wy-IpGR916o&list=TLGQaXtuokbNs&index=12 附氣貼背照片,速治高爾夫球肘(肘隧道症)其他腱鞘炎如腕管綜合症, 踝管綜合症 (腳踭內側痛),拇指側手腕痛(俗稱媽媽手)腱鞘炎 ,扳機指治法的介紹

第 8 篇文章

治網球肘: 網球肘綜合療法

"https://www.youtube.com/watch?v=Wy-IpGR916o&list=TLGQaXtuokbNs&index=12 附氣貼背照片,速治高爾夫球肘(肘隧道症)其他腱鞘炎如腕管綜合症, 踝管綜合症 (腳踭內側痛),拇指側手腕痛(俗稱媽媽手)腱鞘炎 ,扳機指治法的介紹

第 9 篇文章治足前掌痛:

足前掌痛(Morton's neuroma)莫頓氏神經瘤的非手術非藥物療法

https://www.youtube.com/watch?v=0eOjCH4eUQw

第 10 篇文章

https://www.youtube.com/watch?v=abLW9AwVZRc

(粵)行禪唱誦壽而康又名跑步機之山羊太極丹田法 by Dr. George Ho

第 11 篇文章

浮鯨太極速成法 dolphin instant tai chi

https://www.youtube.com/watch?v=vyVey_rJLLU

Other self-published books and articles:
 - MRTC (Med Rehab Tai Chi)
- Dolphin Instant Tai Chi
- Treadmill Ram Tai Chi
-Joint and Related Problems of the Extremities (Hand and leg)
- People's Medicine (1): The Inspirational Case of Bill Clinton's Cure of his Heart Disease
- People's Medicine (2): Plantar Fasciitis
- People's Medicine (3) The Innovative Diagnosis and Treatment Combined Drugless and Non-surgical Therapy of Sacroiliac Joint Dysfunction
- People's Medicine (4) The Rejuvenation Manual (The Heart Rejuvenation Section);
- People's Medicine (5): Wrist Pain of the Ulna (pinky) Side
- Treatment of Tennis Elbow, a Comprehensive Approach

**Profile of Dr. George Kam Wing Ho,
B. Soc. Sc., M.A., D.C.**
Contacts: Georgekwho@yahoo.com
Facebook: http://www.facebook.com/georgekwho

YouTube: Uploads are accessible by keying in "Dr George Ho of Vancouver". Many of my videos will appear.

Skype ID: Georgekwho in Vancouver Canada

Vancouver Research and Teaching Clinic: 5291 Hummingbird Drive, Richmond, B.C. V7E 5T7, Ph. 778-840-4153

Working Experiences

-Associate at the chiropractic clinic of Dr. Ng Shu Yan in Hong Kong<ngshuyanhcc@gmail.com>, 1984-1985

-Registered member of the College of Chiropractors of B C
(http://www.bcchiro.com/)1985-2011

- Health columnist at a Hong Kong magazine, the Financial Trend (the publisher has closed down in 2007.)   1989-2006

-Director of Rehab Tai Chi Program and Honorary Medical Advisor of Vitality Tai Chi Academy, Ref. Tai Chi Master, Mr. Frankie Choi, email: "frankie choi" <funkien@telus.net>   1998- Present

-Registered chiropractor of Hong Kong Government Chiropractic Council, registered#CC000091 2006 till present
(http://www.chiro-council.org.hk/english/index_reg.htm);

- Finished an ergonomic project for the Canadian Consulate of Hong Kong. Reference available on request.   Jan 2008

-Being appointed as an Honorary Medical Advisor of 養生學會, Ref. Louis Tong,
Director（www.islt.com.hk）

- Being invited as a guest speaker at Prof. Ceng-hua Long's lecture on the vertebrogenic origins of organic diseases at Stanford University
Oct., 25,2009
Reference: Prof. Ceng-hua Long, cenghua long longcenghua@163.com (inquiry only in simplified Chinese please)   July 2008 – Present

-Presentation of an academic paper with Prof. Lorenz of Kent State University, "Dantian Singing in Cantonese: A Theory about the Health Impact of Sound" at the Sixth International Conference on Health, Wellness and Society on 21st Oct., 2016 in Washington D.C.
Please compare the following two pictures. In the 2016 picture Dr. Ho appeared younger than the 2009 one. It might be due to his rejuvenation practices.

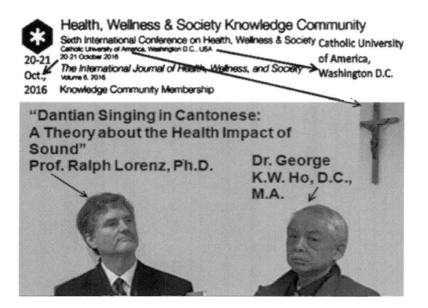

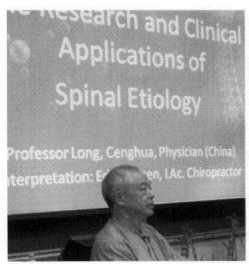

<-Dr. George Ho was invited as a guest speaker at Prof. Ceng-hua Long's lecture on the vertebrogenic origins of organic diseases at Stanford University Oct., 25,2009

41256977R00087

Printed in Poland
by Amazon Fulfillment
Poland Sp. z o.o., Wrocław